Osteogenic Loading

A New Modality To Facilitate Bone Density Development

John Jaquish, Ph.D.

Raj Singh, M.D.

Eleanor Hynote, M.D.

Jason Conviser, Ph.D.

Edited by Lana Denison

Credits:
Chapter 1, 2 adapted from Scott Hopson, Jason Conviser, and Guus van der Meer, Handbook of Acceleration Training: Science, Principles, and Benefits, P.7-22, Copyright © 2007 Power Plate International with permission.

Questions related to the contents to this book should be forwarded to: Jaquish@osteogenic.org
Future updates, and news will be posted on Osteogenic.org

TABLE OF CONTENTS

DEDICATION

Dedicated to my parents Paul and Marie-Jeanne Jaquish. My Father who gave of his time and mechanical engineering talents to help in both prototyping and developing the device described in this book. And my Mother for being the first female test subject to trust me when I had her self-impose over 650 lbs. on her lower extremities in her first osteogenic loading movements.

TABLES AND FIGURES

Figure A-1, bioDensity user interface
Figure A-2, Napa Test Facility authorization to release medical information

FOREWORD

After years of practicing primary care, I became disillusioned with the traditional practice of medicine and began looking for an integrated approach. I felt that traditional practice was focused on "sickness treatment," instead of wellness treatment or prevention. Changing the way I took care of patients to a more preventive type of practice enabled me to research and speak on topics like nutrition, natural medicine, and women's health. This pursuit of knowledge brought me to meet John Jaquish, Ph.D., who had developed and was continuing to refine a device that had great promise, the bioDensity device.

This device provided osteogenic loading and stimulated the neuro-musculoskeletal system to facilitate the natural processes of bone density development, muscular development, and greater nervous system recruitment of tissue in movement. The principles of this bioDensity device were based on published research of mechano-transduction, meaning that loading of the body creates an adaptive response. This research had existed for over 100 years. The cleverness of the device was the level of loading the individual was able to receive while in a safe and controlled environment.

Once learning about this device, I not only prescribed patients exercise/therapy sessions with it, but I also engaged in the use of the device myself. My personal use saw an increase in spinal density and maintenance in hip density within normal T-score range. The spine was osteopenic and was less so after bioDensity use. Equally important was that my full body force production capability increased by 169% in the eight months of using the osteogenic loading protocol, just one time, either weekly or bi-weekly. Since this initial experience I have seen other positive bone mass density outcomes with the use of this device, which are detailed in this book, and I am excited to share my experience so other practitioners like me can use this knowledge with their patients. The discussion in this book will bring to light both the understanding of loading of the body to high degrees and the way this loading takes place in the safe, controlled environment the device provides.

Eleanor Hynote, M.D.
President of the American College for the Advancement of Medicine
Medical Director for Phoenix Wellcare

ABOUT THE AUTHORS

John Jaquish, Ph.D.

John Jaquish is the Chief Technology Officer of Performance Health Systems, and the inventor of both the bioDensity device and its Application Service Provider system network functionality. Dr. Jaquish, after completing many years of research on osteogenic and myofibril function/response, developed the initial prototype of the bioDensity device. Jaquish then conducted four years of testing with human subjects looking at user comfort, biomechanics, and optimal bone and muscular stimulation for individuals from high performance athletics, to the deconditioned and elderly populations. His background in software development enabled him to create a server network that captures and analyzes all usage from bioDensity devices from around the world, providing for the largest known and fastest growing database of physical loading data. Dr. Jaquish holds a holds a Ph.D. in Biomedical Engineering Research from Rushmore University, an MBA from the University of Phoenix, and a BS in Business Administration from California State University. He has been granted five patents for the bioDensity device and global network system by the US Patent and Trademark Office, as well as 222 corresponding international patents in 41 countries.

Raj Singh, M.D.

As the Medical Director for both the Barrow Neurosurgical Associates Diagnostic and Treatment Center and the Rehabilitation Institute of Scottsdale, Dr. Singh is well acquainted with the power of rehabilitative medicine and is considered to be a preeminent specialist in the field of spinal medicine. He is the former Medical Director of the Outpatient Rehabilitation and Spine Program at Barrow Neurological Institute. Dr. Singh also serves as the neurology/rehabilitation consulting physician for the Arizona Diamondbacks team physicians.

Dr. Singh Graduated from Northwestern university medical school and the Rehabilitation Institute of Chicago after completing residency in Neurology, Physical Medicine and Rehabilitation. He is Medical Director of The Barrow Neurosurgical Associates Neurospine and Rehabilitation programs in Phoenix and Scottsdale. He is Board Certified and a Fellow of the American Academy of Physical Medicine & Rehab and The American Association of Neuromuscular and Electro diagnostic Medicine. Dr. Singh is also a Neurosurgical Residency faculty member at Barrow Neurological Institute.

Eleanor Hynote, M.D.

Dr. Hynote is a board-certified internist, and is the Founder and current Director of Phoenix Well Care (PWC) since 1998. A Vassar graduate, Dr. Hynote received her M.D. from The University of California at Irvine, completed her residency training at The California Pacific Medical Center in San Francisco, and completed a fellowship in clinical nutrition and metabolism from The University of California at Davis. Dr. Hynote has logged in thousands of hours of continuing education in both traditional and alternative health care. Notably, she participated in the first training group in Botanical Medicine at Columbia University with Andrew Weil M.D. Dr. Hynote practiced as a primary care physician for nearly a decade and eventually found traditional western medicine practice limiting. Dr. Hynote mentors physicians interested in integrative medicine practice by providing on-site training and ongoing consultation. She is a board member, and 2011 President of the American College for Advancement in Medicine (ACAM), a national organization of over 600 hundred complementary, alternative and integrative physicians. For the past two years, she has served as Program Director for the ACAM biannual conference, which attracts physicians from all over the country.

Jason Conviser, Ph.D.

Jason Conviser is President of JMC & Associates and is one of the country's experts in articulating an opportunity where the traditional health care continuum and health care services are expected and offered in a non-clinical fitness center. Throughout his career, Dr. Conviser has lectured and written about the relationship between exercise and health. Dr. Conviser holds a Ph.D. from the University of Wisconsin and an MBA from Northwestern's Kellogg Graduate School of Business. He is a Fellow of the American College of Sports Medicine.

INTRODUCTION

For the past century the medical community has addressed osteoporosis as an inevitable part of the aging process. Technology developed over the past eight years may mandate the medical community reevaluate their position on this disease state.

This technology enables osteogenic loading, meaning the growth of new bone mass through axial loading of the musculoskeletal system. This new modality for therapy and exercise is a simple and effective intervention that can be widely, safely, and prescribed for many populations. In addition to improving strength and bone health, subjects using osteogenic loading have greatly increased force production, thereby creating the ability to increase balance. The principals of osteogenic loading relate to loading at the levels of high impact exercise. Impact is the stimulation that enables bone mass density as well as muscular density to develop in childhood, these loads are multiples of bodyweight, loading levels far higher than any found in fitness. In adulthood these benefits can be seen in high impact activity such as gymnastics with above normal bone mass density and incredible power-to-weight ratio, but injury risk makes this activity undesirable for most adults.

This book is about how adults can replicate the bone and muscular benefits from the "childhood impact behavior." Beginning with a basic understanding of what systems this modality stimulates is important, therefore this book starts with chapters that highlight both bone and muscular tissues, their function, and adaptations to the impact stimulus that is being created with osteogenic loading. For those who fully understand bone and muscular function, some chapters can be skipped. Please note the table of contents.

Definition:
bioDensity - The first device application of osteogenic loading principals.

In this book we will discuss the relationships of strength, and bone health in relation to ostengenic loading. We will explore the processes of bone remodeling and the prevention/treatment of osteoporosis, and we will examine the concepts at work as osteogenic loading improves bone density in thousands of people around the world.

CHAPTER 1

GROSS STRUCTURE AND

FUNCTION OF BONE

What is Bone Tissue?

The skeletal framework of the body bears mechanical loading of movement, moves the body via muscular attachment, and supports the organs of the body. Bone (our skeletal framework) is an amazing tissue. It can be as strong as metal while as light as wood. When a bone fracture occurs the healing process begins almost immediately. Bone mass also acts like a battery, storing calcium and phosphorus, which are required for many cellular functions throughout the body. The loss of an individual's bone mass can impact other organs and functions of the body, as nutrients required for function may not be present from the lack of bone mass. Osteoporosis and its precursor, osteopenia are determined by the lack of axial mechanical loading over time. Typically this is affiliated with aging and other age related disease states. However, younger individuals are susceptible as well if proper loading is not applied to bone mass.

When action potential (signal from the brain to physically move) from the central nervous system is applied to muscular tissue, mechanical loading is placed on the bone mass. The tension, compression, and torsion being placed on the bone mass, with the proper level of loading, can have an osteogenic effect. This means that at certain levels of mechanical loading, bone mass density can be increased. These levels can be varied based on the condition of the individual, for example an osteoporotic individual may respond to lower axial mechanical loading than an individual within normal bone mass.

Definition: Osteoblasts - Bone cells responsible for forming and depositing new bone matrix. Following bone fractures osteoclasts and osteoblasts play important roles in repair. There is a delicate balance that must be maintained between these two cell types. If osteoclasts remove old tissue too fast, there is a net bone loss.

Definition: Osteoclasts - Bone cells charged with resorbing bone matrix by dissolving its calcium and phosphate, and releasing it into the bloodstream. Osteoclasts create an acidic microenvironment that is necessary to dissolve bone minerals and to activate the enzymes to break down collagen fibers.

Bone has several components, each having different functions. The compact tissue is the most important for the strength of the bone. This is the outer shell and the hardest part of the bone. This layer is being remodeled from the inside out, with osteoblasts that "grab" minerals based on axial mechanical loading falling in this hard layer underneath the older osteoblasts that meet osteoclasts at the surface. The osteoclasts then degrade the older bone mass so the minerals can be used in other functions of the body. Many osteoporosis medications focus on retarding this natural process of shedding the older bone, which some researchers suggest is related to many of the side effects of these drugs.

This hardened tissue forms canals that run along the axis of the bone to encase capillaries and nerve fibers, these canal structures are called, Haversian Canals. Inside of the hardened shell is the medullary cavity, containing cancellous tissue. This is the softer tissue that often holds bone marrow.

There are three types of bone tissue:

1. Compact tissue - This outer layer of the bone is the hardest and most dense part of the bone. This outer part of bone tissue is arranged in canals or tube-like structures called Haversian canals, which run parallel to the long axis of the bone. These hardened structures have capillaries and nerve fibers within them.

2. Cancellous tissue - This is the sponge-like tissue inside the medullary cavity of the bone, where the bone marrow is located.

3. Subchondral tissue - This is the smooth tissue that is protected by cartilage, at the ends of the bones.

Force and Bone

When force is applied to bone mass, in a compressive, bending, torsion or stretching manner, the cellular response can cause an adaptation for the bones to potentially grow, provided the loading attains the proper osteogenic level. The weight of bone per volume (usually reflected in grams/cm squared) is the measure of bone mass density.

Bone is not just a mechanical lever supporting movement. Bone tissue also performs metabolic functions, storing 99% of the body's calcium and 85% of the body's phosphorous. The body's tight range of healthy blood calcium is regulated by hormones, and when necessary, the body will remove calcium from bones to meet its needs elsewhere.

Water comprises 25% of adult health bone matrix. The weight of mineral per volume of bone is referred to as Bone Mineral Density (BMD). Bone Mineral Density can be measured, and many individuals take this test after age 50 to be forewarned about loss of bone strength.

Physical Strength and Healthy Bone

Recent research shows that physical activity at a young age predisposes people to the benefits of healthy bones in later years. Even if the subjects no longer do exercise training, their bone density is better than if they had not trained earlier in their lives.

Since the early days of space exploration, axial mechanical loading has played a role in counteracting the effects of microgravity. While away from Earth's gravity, astronauts are subjected to unloaded states: their muscles, tendons, and bones are not required to resist gravity and do not need to work. Under these conditions, astronauts lose bone density at alarming rates. Patients confined to bed rest suffer similar effects from the lack of mechanical loading they experience. Microgravity influences the body's capacity to maintain orthostatic (fainting) tolerance and its ability to perform physical exercise. It causes an early reduction in blood volume and subsequent loss of red blood cell volume, resulting in limited cardiac filling. There is also evidence that cardiovascular structures become altered during microgravity, which may cause cardiac atrophy.

Other consequences of the lack of loading on the musculoskeletal system include alterations in the structure and function of vascular smooth muscle. Vascular smooth muscle contraction is reduced, causing altered morphology, or atrophy, and lower vaso-reactivity. Lung function is also affected in simulated microgravity or bed rest due to the lack of loading on the musculoskeletal system. Bed rest does not affect lungs as adversely as spaceflight does, but the muscular system is adversely affected because the skeleton is unloaded, and respiratory muscles are unused.

The overall result of such microgravity is a degradation of the body's capacity to generate force and a reduced capacity for oxygen delivery to the muscle cells. Astronauts in space and patients confined to bed both suffer from the effects of microgravity (or less than normal gravity).

Extended bed rest is simulated microgravity, and may cause loss of bone within three weeks of sustained inaction. The state of microgravity affects the human body through several mechanisms, one of which is atrophy, or tissue wasting from the lack of loading of the body. In this state body fluids redistribute and cause the baroreceptors, which regulate blood pressure, to lose responsiveness. Decrease in muscle mass and loss of strength can occur after just 2 weeks in bed. In 6 weeks, the heart muscle, or cardiac mass, is decreased, and in 12 weeks, bone mineral density may show a decrease (Leblanc, et al. 2009).

Muscle atrophy is expressed by the reduced cross-section of muscle fibers. Fast-twitch muscle fibers lose more size than slow-twitch fibers. In addition, the patient may experience negative changes in muscle morphology, such as edema, disrupted myofibrils, and striation, and activities of enzymes related to metabolic pathways are altered.

Bone Remodelling

Human bones are dynamic organs, not just static structures supporting the body. Bone has been described as resembling reinforced concrete: its hard calcium phosphate matrix is inflexible and is reinforced by flexible fibers of collagen, a protein that plays a role similar to steel reinforcement bars. Under the surface, most bone looks like a rigid sponge or a meshwork of tissue. This works and acts like the framing of a building; inside there are regularly spaced studs, allowing flow and supporting the structure while minimizing weight.

Bone is efficient and responds to functional demands and muscle attachments with bone remodeling. In remodeling, bone is removed where it is not required and added where needed. Bone dynamics consist of continual resorption (tearing down) and formation (building up) of bone matrix. There is a constant information exchange in the body, along with continual bone tissue renovation that removes existing bone and deposits new bone. In the first year of life, the skeleton will replace 100% of itself. A young adult's skeleton will replace 20% of its bone tissue each year. Once bone has stopped forming, around the age of 28, peak bone mass is maintained by a process of remodeling. Bone tissue has a slow turnover rate, as the cycle of remodeling is between 3 to 4 months and between 6 to 8 months (Mundy, 1999) for the mineralization to be noticed with the current DXA scanning technology that is used today. Tomorrow's new bone cells reflect the quality of your efforts today.

Bone remodelling is constant, and hormones control this continuous process. Resorption, the teardown process performed by osteoclasts, and remodelling happens with the action of osteoblasts. If osteoclasts outpace osteoblasts, bone loses density. For example, after women pass the age of 30, bone resorption may begin to outpace bone formation. After menopause, usually between the ages of 45-55, the risk of osteoporosis increases to the point that women can lose up to 3% to 5% BMD per year.

While osteoclastic and osteoblastic functions are both encouraged during high levels of axial musculoskeletal loading, most drug intervention programs work on inhibiting the osteoclasts without addressing osteoblastic activity. Drugs can therefore be considered ineffective long-term solutions and may potentially hinder normal bone remodelling.

Bone is alive! There are three types of living cells that receive blood from crisscrossing vessels. The dense cellular matrix and blood supply enable bone to constantly rebuild on a microscopic level while remaining stable at a macroscropic level. While the exterior may appear to be solid, this compact-looking bone is just a shell.

Bone Remodeling, Cells, and Their Functions

breathing and lowering chance of injury in the future.

Bone Density Increases

Forces that briefly bend or compress bones stimulate an adaptive response of bone density growth (Wolff, 1892, U.S. Surgeon General, 2004). This level of force/loading typically requires multiples of an individuals bodyweight (Marcus, 2006). Test subjects produced higher forces than would be seen in conventional fitness environments. bioDensity system collected data (bD server, 2012) demonstrates multiples of bodyweight loading for different populations:

- *Athlete Population - 75th percentile bD Leg Press for males ages 20 to 29 (n=279) is 2,790 lbs./1,268 kg.*

- *Adult Population - 50th percentile bD Leg Press for males ages 40 to 49 (n=380) is 2,031 lbs./923 kg.*

- *Aging Population - 50th percentile bD Leg Press for females ages 80 to 99 (n=142) is 635 lbs./289 kg.*

The test subjects above had adapted up to these levels of force over 48 bD sessions. Clinical research (n=4,374) has shown force production improvements averaging 6.1% in females and 5.1% in males between sessions 3 and 4 (Moynes et al. 2013). Both the levels of force used and gains in force production capability have corresponded with increases in bone density verified by DXA scans (Jaquish et al. 2012).

Benjamin, M. Ralphs, J. (1998). Fibrocartilage in tendons and ligaments - an adaptation to compressive load. Journal of Anatomy. 9:481–494.

bioDensity Server Query (2012). Users/Patients from worldwide bioDensity network, 132 locations surveyed. Data prerequisites include, completion of face sheet questionnaire and up to 48 bD uses.

Hebb, D. (1949). *The Organization of Behavior: A Neuropsychological Theory.* New York, NY: Wiley.

Jaquish, J.; Singh, R. Hynote, E. Conviser, J. (2012), *Osteogenic Loading.* Nevada City, CA: JIR.

Kraemer, William J.; Zatsiorsky, Vladimir M. (2006). *Science and practice of strength training.* Champaign, IL: Human Kinetics. p.50.

Marcus, R. (1996) Skeletal Impact of Exercise. The Lancet. November 1996. 384(9038); 1326-1327.

Mookerjee, S. Ratamess, N. (1999). "Comparison of Strength Differences and Joint Action Durations Between Full and Partial Range-of-Motion Bench Press Exercise. Journal of Strength and Conditioning Research, 1999, 13(1), 76–81 National Strength & Conditioning Association.

Moynes, R. Smith, D. Rockey, S. Conviser, J. & Skinner, J. (2013, May). bioDensity™ Training: Methodology, use, and quantification of baseline strength. Presented at the annual meeting of the ACSM, Indianapolis, Indiana.

U.S. Surgeon General (2004). Bone health and osteoporosis: a report of the Surgeon General. Rockville, Md.: U.S. Dept. of Health and Human Services, Public Health Service, Office of the Surgeon General; Washington, D.C.: U.S. G.P.O., 2004. p.223.

Wolff J. (1892). The Law of Bone Remodeling. Berlin Heidelberg New York: Springer, (Marquet and Furlong, 1986 translation of the German 1892 edition).

bioDensity™

bioDensity™ Force Production Increase: Clinical Analysis with Over 4,000 Subjects

Force production is the metric that bioDenstiy (bD) uses to measure both stimulus and changes in the body. Increases in force production have been seen by researchers in more than 4,000 test subjects as presented at the American College of Sports Medicine annual conference (Moynes et al. 2013). This paper discusses various human body adaptations resulting from this increase.

Broad Population Benefits

Increasing bone density, greater activation of the central nervous system, and improving the strength and alignment of joints are benefits that improve lives of high performance athletes as well as deconditioned, compromised and elderly individuals. bD use can deliver these positive changes to the body, and do so safely as all forces applied are regulated by the patient/user's own comfort. As a result injuries (and falls) can be reduced/prevented and performance (in athletics or in every day life) improves.

- Safe - All force/load is self imposed
- Accurate & repeatable - Server based ensuring the same experience in all locations

Neurological Amplification

The bD system isolates optimal biomechanical positions, allowing the greatest amount of tissue activation. These positions have been identified through analysis of force production and motor neuron engagement (Mookerjee & Ratamess, 1999). When an individual engages large amounts muscular cells in action, the cells work together more effectively over time (Hebb, 1949). Motor learning, begins this way and as the individual repeats and speeds the action, greater neural adaptive responses take place. Rapid neurological changes take place upon the first 4 uses of bD as identified by researchers showing full body force production gains of 9.3% between second and third sessions of bD (Moynes et al. 2013).

Stronger Joints, Reinforced Connective Tissue, and Improved Biomechanics

Similar to bone, compressive forces also improve the density of tendons and ligaments. This reinforcement of tendons and ligaments dissipates stress at joints allowing for greater performance and less pain in movement (Benjamin & Ralphs, 1998). This means bone can realign to

Elastic strength is the ability of the neuromuscular system to switch quickly and efficiently from an eccentric contraction or a muscle lengthening contraction, to a concentric contraction or muscle shortening contraction.

Endurance strength is the ability to produce and maintain force over prolonged periods of time.

Speed strength, or power, is the ability of the neuromuscular system to produce the greatest possible force in the shortest possible time.

Stability strength, or balance?, is the ability of the kinetic chain's stabilizing muscles to provide optimal dynamic joint stabilization and maintain postural equilibrium during functional movements.

Functional strength is the ideal level of strength that an individual requires to perform activity-specific functional movements.

Core strength is the ability of the musculature of the torso, spine, and lumbo-pelvic-hip complex to control an individual's constantly changing center of gravity.

Strength and Power

All of life's functional movements require diverse applications of force at varied speeds and timing, and all of us need the skills of speed and force to produce each of those movements. For example, we are all vulnerable to unstable environments (even a trained athlete can slip on a patch of ice). Each individual requires sufficient balance and stability for life's daily activities, such as a reserve of neuromuscular power to prevent falling. People also need strength in order to function fully in life.

To perform their best, athletes require each of the elements of strength and power in order. Training for power is a priority for many athletes, which is a challenge because phases and cycles of periodized training must be carefully planned to encourage ultimate in-season performance. All components of strength—such as power, stability, endurance, and balance—vary in application and time under tension but are still considered "force."

Training specificity and the intent of training are the most important factors in achieving specific goals. Training for explosive power must include movements that activate the stretch reflex in preparation for the movement, a concept called the stretch-shortening cycle. Skills and movements must be trained according to the Specific Adaptations to Imposed Demands of the sport or activity (the S.A.I.D. principle). A major advantage to employing osteogenic loading is that it allows individuals to generate more force with higher loads.

CHAPTER 3

NEURAL CONTROL OF MUSCLE

CONTRACTION

The central nervous system (CNS) controls the contraction of a given skeletal muscle. Skeletal muscle differs from smooth and cardiac muscle, both of which can contract without being stimulated by the CNS. The following is a general overview of the CNS function with muscular contraction.

The neuro-motor system is organized into two major parts. The CNS consists of (1) the brain and spinal cord and (2) the peripheral nervous systems (PNS). Which consists of nerves that supply information to and from the CNS. The intentional action during a complex learned movement, such as a golf swing, involves a chain of neuromuscular patterns, not simply muscular strength. Millions of bits of information are processed by the CNS mechanisms in nervous system control mechanisms. The input and responses optimize and increase efficiency as an individual develops skeletal muscle and learned motor patterns.

The Brain and Motor Function

The adult human brain weighs about three pounds. It is divided into three parts:
1. Brainstem, an extension of the spinal cord.
2. Cerebellum.
3. Forebrain, primarily the cerebrum.

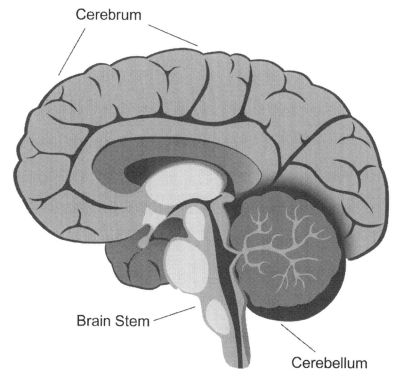

Cerebrum

Brain Stem

Cerebellum

Figure 3-1, Major parts of the brain

The forebrain and cerebellum are divided into two separated hemispheres that are connected by a band of nerve fibers. The hemispheres have "lobes," which perform specific functions. For example, muscular control takes place in the motor cortex located in the frontal lobe.

Two kinds of nerve fibers—axons and dendrites—which make up a nerve cell, also called a neuron. These both protrude from the center of most neurons. A neuron typically has numerous dendrites and one axon.

Dendrites

In most neurons, the dendrite fibers are relatively short and highly branched' they function as the communication links to other neurons. The dendrites themselves have tiny, thorn-like spines on their surfaces, which serve as contact points for parts of other neurons.

Axons

Axons are long fibers of a neuron that act somewhat similar to a fiber-optic cable carrying one-way messages to tissue. A neuron sends electrical impulses through the axon to the target cells it controls. The axon terminal is the point where the electrical signal sent from one neuron to another is changed into a chemical signal to be sent to the next neuron.

Neuromuscular junctions (synapses) are the contact point where a motor neuron connects to a muscle. After traveling down the motor neurons of the sensory-somatic branch of the nervous system, nerve impulses cause the contraction of the skeletal muscle fibers at which they terminate. Acetylcholine, (a neurotransmitter that facilitates skeletal muscle contraction) is released from the axon terminal when an nerve impulse reaches the junction. Chemical changes cross the synapse and stimulate the formation of an electrical impulse, which is produced in the muscle cell when the activating element binds to the receptors. Calcium, which is stored in the cells, is released by the impulse, which causes a single, short muscle contraction called a twitch.

Skeletal muscle is organized into hundreds of motor units, each of which involves a motor neuron, connected by the long axons. These attach to and control specific groups of muscle fibers. A conditioned response to specific circumstance will determine the precise number of motor units used. With a complete contraction, each motor unit is still independent but can work with all other motor units for combined strength and coordination. Motor unit recruitment depends on need. When an individual loses balance and must brace for impact of the upper extremities with the ground, the contraction will engage a far greater amount of motor units than getting up off of the ground by using the upper extremities. This is a comparison of need by looking at the mechanical loading required, the impact being multiples of bodyweight, and the "getting up" action being a fraction of bodyweight.

Tetanus

The process of contracting takes approximately 50 milliseconds, and relaxation of the fiber takes another 50 to 100 msec. Because the refractory period is so much shorter than the time needed for contraction and relaxation, the muscle fiber can be maintained in the contracted state as long as the action potential stimulus remains, this is when a muscle contracts, and can not release either by conscious or subconscious process. Such sustained contraction is called tetanus.

Neurological Implication of Loading

Mechanical loading of the body can cause neural adaptation: the body learns movement and awakens neuromuscular pathways, and function improves over time. There is a reciprocal inhibition of the opposing muscles (the functional antagonists) and the assisting muscles (the synergists). The neural pathway at work is called a polysynaptic pathway, which is the mechanism responsible for simultaneous gains in flexibility and strength. Neural adaptation also encompasses intramuscular coordination and an increased firing rate of motor units.

Sensory-Motor Factors, Proprioception and Reflexes

Sensory motor adaptation describes the stimulation of nervous system receptors and assists in heightening neuromuscular capacity, which has a positive influence on force production. Vibration after enhanced neuromuscular performance is related to an increased sensitivity of the stretch reflex. However, it is important to note that Golgi Tendon Organs, joints also perceive impact-level mechanical loading. This results in further improvements in flexibility, joint stabilization, sensory motor feedback and body awareness. The sensory motion feedback is also called proprioception.

The body reflexively provides the expertise to recruit and coordinate strength and power for intense physical activity, such as fight-or-flight situations or intense exercise. Stimulation above and beyond normal exercise loads, such as impact-level loading, causes the neuromuscular system to recruit and coordinate the greatest number of movement pathways, including more muscle and nerve fibers. Stimulation of underutilized pathways helps coordinate a greater capacity for movement and allows the body to perform at higher levels.

CHAPTER 4

MUSCLE AND

BONE STRENGTH

Muscle and bone have a synergistic relationship. In the process of development, a muscle becomes stronger and can apply greater loads on the skeletal system, which in part creates greater bone density. The stronger and less porous the bone tissue becomes, the more the integrity and function of the skeletal muscular system is enhanced. As bone mass density increases, an individual will become more capable of managing higher loads over time. This adaptation of both muscle and bone tissue occurs as both an acute and chronic response, with the benefits of neuromuscular re-education and motor pattern reinforcement. The overall effect creates movement efficiency and skill, impacting every system in the body required for the production of force: the neural system and the physiological, mechanical, metabolic, and hormonal systems.

Osteogenic loading allows multiple benefits to be realized simultaneously. Improvement is seen in strength and power, muscle tone, and aesthetics, with improved circulation, better bone density, pain reduction, anabolic hormone production, increased oxygen delivery, boosted metabolism, and improved recovery. This loading enhances muscle recruitment so that a high percentage of all muscle fibers are engaged, including activation of joint stabilizer and core muscles, which promotes joint health and core stability.

Use of osteogenic loading enhances strength and reverses weaknesses caused by inactivity. Because the benefits are so versatile and comprehensive, the use of osteogenic loading provides the tools to improve numerous deficits. Most individuals can attribute their strengths to their specific training programs, and their unaddressed needs may remain neglected. The application of osteogenic loading offers a solution to these deficits, with inclusive, fast, and simple health solutions.

While not every individual needs every physical skill, to remain healthy and adaptable we all need strength, power, endurance, sensory motor feedback, coordination, bone density, and good recovery. Using osteogenic loading, competitive lifters can enhance their potential by means of increased muscle activation and speed while maintaining absolute strength. Elite athletes can stay strong and fast and can also develop a higher power-to-weight ratio without the risk of injury. Endurance athletes wishing to improve strength, speed, power, and recovery can achieve all of their goals using osteogenic loading and without compromising endurance.

The Adaptive Response of Muscular Tissue

For an active individual, the process of imposing progressively higher loads on the skeletal muscle tissue results in increased muscle performance and size. This is called muscular hypertrophy, and it happens in two ways:

1. Sarcoplasmic Development - As detailed by Zatsiorsky (2006) in *Science and Practice of Strength Training*, "sarcoplasmic hypertrophy of muscle fibers is characterized by the growth of sarcoplasm (semifluid interfibrillar substance) and non-contractile proteins

that do not directly contribute to the production of muscle force." Sarcoplasmic hypertrophy occurs when an individual engages in physical movement with load applied. This could be lifting weights or, to a lesser degree, walking (p.67). An increase of sarcoplasm, the fluid kept within the cell, with little change in actual functional performance of the cell, allows for greater muscular function. Consisting of glycogen, proteins, and other components, this fluid stays within the cell for only a matter days depending on diet, sleep, and conditioning (Kreitzman et al., 1992). Individuals who engage in exercise in order to enlarge muscular cells as much as possible are primarily creating a sarcoplasmic effect. Of activities that induce this type of muscular adaptation, the most common adaptive response to exercising includes lifting conventional weights selected to enable multiple repetitions, commonly the 10 to 12 repetition range. The action of creating this adaptation provides greater circulation for a brief period of time, as well as an increase in cardiovascular demand. During these repetitions blood is being shunted to the contracting muscles involved in the motor movement, which then delivers oxygen to the cells. Blood also carries glycogen and proteins, some of which stay behind after the blood leaves the target muscle group or groups. This sarcoplasmic development may have a compounding effect as the individual exercises over weeks and months. However, after a given period of time, muscle cells will have enlarged to the point where they reach the maximum amount of sarcoplasm, and continued efforts will have diminishing returns. This is seen with individuals who begin an exercise program and progress rapidly, but eventually stop progressing. Additional strength is built through this process by virtue of additional glycogen being held within the cell, which over this period of time enables the cells to respond to higher energy demand on the body. This higher energy demand, coming from the act of engaging both the muscle with enlarged cells and the resting muscle, manifests itself as a higher metabolic rate (Kreitzman et al., 1992). Unfortunately, when an individual must take a break from exercising (for injury, vacation, or whatever reason), this sarcoplasm begins to dissipate, sometimes in a week or 10 days (McGuff, 2003).

2. Myofibril Development - An increase in the thickness of the individual fibers due to an increase in the amount of myofibrils within sarcomere structures, an adaptive response that enables greater force production from muscular tissue. The myofibrils are formed as a result of a CNS stimulus of momentary muscular failure. This means stopping the performance of an exercise from fatigue. The free-floating proteins within the sarcoplasm combine as actin and myosin in sarcomere structures. This myofibril stimulus requires momentary muscular failure under maximal loads.

From a long-term health perspective this is a greater adaptive response as this functional strength applies to all activities of daily living, as well as the synergy of building and maintaining strength in order to continue to build and maintain greater balance and stability. From an athletic perspective, creates a higher power-to-weight ratio and is a far preferred adaptive response for strength and speed creation.

Definition:
Momentary muscular failure - An occurrence where an individual engaging in an exercise reaches a point in a repetition of the exercise where the target muscles can no longer contract. Most occurrences of momentary muscular failure involve the

expenditure of stored energy units (ATP, glycogen, and creatine phosphate), which yield a sarcoplasmic adaptation. When momentary muscular failure occurs due to a mechanical inability to produce or withstand additional load, a myofibril adaptation can be achieved.

Myofibril Development and Bone Strength

When children play, they often run and jump and sometimes fall down. This impact stimulus on their bodies is, as described in the jump-training analysis paper (Marcus, 1996), a far larger load than that of their own body weight. This increases both their bone mass and, in a specific way, their muscular mass. The loads they are receiving are not necessarily repetitive; therefore, they do not resemble the exercise model presented above. Instead, these loads stimulate myofibril development. The running, jumping, and the general mechanical impact loading on a child's body eventually evolves into a less active behavior pattern. Myofibril development can continue in explosive fashion in an athletic individual who is using weights, and doing other athletic activities. Obviously, this means that very few individuals will receive the stimulus for myofibril development beyond childhood or young adulthood if they do not participate in high-impact activity.

From the perspective of health, wellness, and athletic performance, myofibril development is one of the variables that needs to be maintained. However, until now there has been no practical way to stimulate this adaptive response due to limitations of conventional training modalities. An individual who can create a great amount of myofibril development can place larger amounts of mechanical loading on the body engine, thereby continuing to positively affect bone mass density. Bone density and muscular performance can be directly related.

The differences between sarcoplasmic and myofibril hypertrophy are shown below:

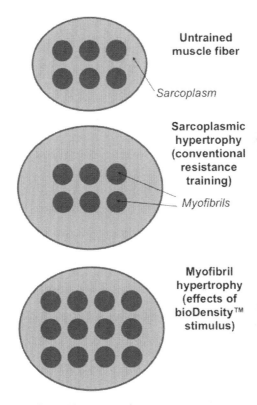

Figure 4-1, Myofibril Hypertrophy

Osteogenic Loading

All of the cells described are necessary for response to damage of the bone tissue, as well as the natural process of generating bone mass density. When a fracture or other damage occurs, the cells call on other bone cells, such as osteoblasts, to begin the repair process. These damage-repair cells will actually force the osteoblasts to migrate to the damaged area and begin to deposit a new collagen matrix that will eventually become mineralized bone tissue.

Ideally, old bone mass is replaced via the osteoclast function with the formation of new bone mass, and a constant density of bone matrix is maintained. When this process does not remain balanced, older bone mass breaks down, but a newer bone mass fails to form. If this happens for just a brief period of time, the bone mass can be brought back to optimal levels, commonly referred to as peak bone mass, which, as discussed in the previous chapter, is attained at the end of puberty. If the balance of bone mass breakdown and repair fails for an extended period of time, osteopenia and eventually osteoporosis will manifest. Up to 90% of an individual's peak bone mass will be determined by age 18 in females, age 20 in males.

Osteogenic loading provides benefits to bone mineral density because of the high levels of axial mechanical loading that are used, interwoven benefits of improved circulation, strength, power, hormone profile, proprioception, balance, and coordination.

Osteogenic loading also works to improve general health and wellness in the following ways:

1. Levels of axial mechanical loading to the skeletal system that approach or match the levels of impact are the most useful for increasing or maintaining bone mass (U.S. Surgeon General, 2004).

2. Loading of the muscular system, at the levels of impact, which are often multiples of body-weight, induce rapid muscular hypertrophy, even after just one use (Mookerjee and Ratamass, 1999).

3. Enhanced coordination and balance occurs because of the body's proprioception and reflexes with added strength, as when an individual is put off balance, there is a greater ability to correct the imbalance with reflexes because of the added strength. This enables greater loading during other activities of daily living.

4. After an osteogenic loading session improved vascular delivery occurs in bone, muscle, connective, and other tissues throughout the body, causing fluid movement and fluid pressure, activating osteogenesis.

6. The combination of these factors provides the benefits of an improved anabolic hormone profile, supporting regeneration and growth of bone tissue.

7. Due to all of these factors, bone regeneration is encouraged, and growth matches or outpaces bone resorption, leading to an increase in bone mineral density.

8. The myofibril muscular hypertrophy that osteogenic loading provides enhances an individual's metabolic rate, potentially advancing fat-loss programs.

A summary of 1-8 suggests, these physiological factors created by osteogenic loading are supported by existing research (some dating back to 1892) showing that the benefits of osteogenic loading support the bone remodeling process in those who need it. At-risk populations enjoy enhanced strength, activation of muscles and tendons, improved circulation, and elevated growth hormone.

CHAPTER 5

OSTEOPOROSIS: DEFINITION, CURRENT TREATMENTS, AND MYTHS

Osteoporosis Definition

Osteoporosis, is the loss of bone mass, with a resulting greater porosity of the bone. This loss occurs from osteoblastic function where the lack of axial mechanical loading (force being placed on the bone tissue) results in new osteoblasts failing to retain minerals, specifically calcium and phosphate. As an osteoblast emerges from the center of the bone, through its migratory process to the outer cortex, the osteoblast will either retain minerals as a response to mechanical loading or migrate without gathering minerals. Low levels of mechanical loading will yield lower mineral retention, thereby lowering the density of the entire bone.

When the process of decreasing bone mass density begins, it is called osteopenia, which is the precursor to osteoporosis. Individuals with either diagnosis may experience the following:

- Bone pain to the touch
- Fractures with minimal stress
- Loss of height (up to 6 inches) over time

- Low back pain due to small fractures of the vertebrae
- Neck pain due to fractures of the vertebrae
- Stooped posture or kyphosis

Osteoporosis   Healthy bone

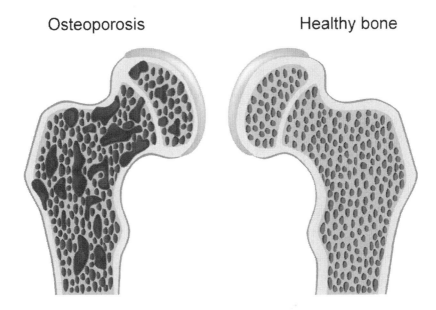

Figure 5-1, Bone mass density development

If left untreated, osteopenia progresses into osteoporosis, in which an even greater bone mass loss is observed, adversely affecting posture and increasing risk of fracture. Most apparent when seeing someone with osteoporosis is the exaggerated spinal curvature. The National Center for Biotechnology Information refers to osteoporotic exaggerated spinal curvature: "The spine weakens with age, becoming more curved and more fragile." (NCBI, 2011).

The following are global osteoporosis facts and statistics from the International Osteoporosis Foundation's publication)

(2010) Facts and Statistics About Osteoporosis and its Impact:

- Osteoporosis affects an estimated 75 million people in Europe, the USA, and Japan.

- For the year 2000, there were an estimated 9 million new osteoporotic fractures, of which 1.6 million were at the hip, 1.7 million were at the forearm, and 1.4 million were clinical vertebral fractures. Europe and the Americas accounted for 51% of all these fractures, while most of the remainder occurred in the Western Pacific region and Southeast Asia.

- 1 in 3 women over 50 will experience osteoporotic fractures, as will 1 in 5 men.

- Nearly 75% of hip, spine and distal forearm fractures occur among patients 65 years old or over.

- A 10% loss of bone mass in the vertebrae can double the risk of vertebral fractures, and similarly, a 10% loss of bone mass in the hip can result in a 2.5 times greater risk of hip fracture.

- By 2050, the worldwide incidence of hip fracture in men is projected to increase by 310% and 240% in women.

- In white women, the lifetime risk of hip fracture is 1 in 6, compared with a 1 in 9 risk of a breast cancer diagnosis.

- In women over 45 years of age, osteoporosis accounts for more days spent in hospital than many other diseases, including diabetes, myocardial infarction, and breast cancer.

- Although low BMD confers increased risk of fracture, most fractures occur in postmenopausal women and elderly men at moderate risk.

Commonly Accepted Risk Factors for Osteoporosis

- Absence of menstrual periods for extended periods of time

- Drinking excess alcohol

- Family history of osteoporosis

- History of hormonal therapy for prostate or breast cancer

- Lower than normal body weight

- Tobacco

- Shortage of calcium in the diet

How is Osteoporosis Detected?

Early detection of osteoporosis requires a bone density test. The most common test is called a central DXA (dual energy x-ray absorptiometry) scan. DXA technology is designed to emit two simultaneous x-ray beams aimed at an individual's hip or spine. The level of absorption of these x-ray beams is used to determine the density of the bone mass. The beams have differing energy levels, thereby distinguishing them from each other. Typically, women over the age of 65 are at higher risk for loss of bone mass and are prime candidates for a DXA scan.

The DXA scan is reported in both, T-scores and Z-scores. The T-score is the number of standard deviations above or below the average for a young adult at peak bone density, but there can be differences based on reference group. The Z-score is a number of standard deviations below an average person of the same age group. Both scores are valuable for the diagnosis of osteoporosis. Another measure of bone mass density is grams per centimeter squared, $(g/cm2)$, which addresses raw volume of bone mass with no normative comparison. The DXA test emits low levels of radiation, is not painful, and requires only five minutes to complete.

Osteoporosis plagues millions of people, and is largely caused by a lack of axial mechanical loading at a level that will stimulate an adaptive response in osteoblasts. Osteoporosis is induced by a lack of load being placed on the body, which is a requirement for bone mineral absorption. While often associated with the aging process, osteoporosis is also seen in demographic groups. Children and young adults suffer from this disease if they are immobilized for one reason or another and are unable to load the body. Astronauts who spend extended periods of time without the benefit of the gravitational pull of the earth also experience osteoporosis. All of these groups can have relative recovery from osteoporosis with the appropriate exercise prescription/dose response. With conventional modalities this process becomes more difficult as individuals age. In a study by Tsuzuku, et al. (2001) bone mass density generation was observed with high-intensity resistance training, but was not effective with low-intensity resistance training. Subjects included males in their 20s as both test and control participants. The results showed increases in bone mass with the test group that was using the heaviest mechanical loading possible on the body, whereas results with the control group showed no change in bone mass.

In a similar study, 14 post-menopausal, osteoporotic women were subjected to loading of the distal forearm (wrist) with high-intensity loads while a control group of was inactive. The baseline DXA tests were done one year prior to the beginning of the study. The loading was applied three times per week for five months. The non-exercising control group averaged a loss of 1.9% bone mass density, whereas the group that received the loading increased bone mass density by 3.8% (Simkin, Avalon, Leichter, 1987).

Medications for Osteoporosis

The following is a list of existing U.S. Food and Drug Administration (FDA) approved medications and their known side effects. Some of the most commonly prescribed osteoporosis drugs are Bisphosphonates.

Bisphosphonates Facts and Risks

These drugs are antiresorptive medicines, which means they slow or stop the natural process that dissolves bone tissue, resulting in maintained or increased bone density and strength (ACOG, 2008). Specifically they stop the process of the osteoclasts. This is the process during which the older osteoblasts are dissolved in favor of the newer osteoblasts that are migrating into the outer cortex, the hard outer layer. The process of the bisphosphonates forces the body to keep the older bone cells, but as bone cells refresh on a six-year basis, eventually this process will falter, as research has shown (Coxon, et al., 2000). The currently prescribed bisphosphonates are alendronate sodium (Fosamax), risendronate (Actonel), ibandronate (Boniva), zoledronic acid (Reclast), and etidronate (Didronel), which is not approved by the FDA for osteoporosis but it is prescribed in Canada and Europe. According to the FDA, side effects of bisphosphonates are the following:

Source: U.S. Food and Drug Administration (2010). Bisphosphonates (marketed as Actonel, Actonel+Ca, Aredia, Boniva, Didronel, Fosamax, Fosamax+D, Reclast, Skelid, and Zometa)

1. Esophagus problems: These problems include irritation, inflammation, or ulcers of the esophagus, which may sometimes bleed.

2. Low calcium levels in the blood (hypocalcemia): Low blood calcium must be treated before an individual can take a Bisphosphonate medication. Most people with low blood calcium levels do not have symptoms, but some people may have symptomsthat include, spasms, twitches, or cramps in the muscles, numbness or tingling in the fingers, toes, or around the mouth.

3. Bone, joint, or muscle pain

4. Severe jaw bone problems (osteonecrosis) The jaw bone begins to lose blood supply. The bones then collapse, leading to pain and arthritis, which can hinder the use of the jaw.

5. Unusual thigh bone fractures

Non-Bisphosphonates Facts and Risks

Raloxifene (Evista) is another osteoporosis medication. The following is the list of side effects found on the FDA website for EVISTA:

"Serious and life-threatening side effects can occur while taking EVISTA. These include blood clots and dying from stroke: Increased risk of blood clots in the legs (deep vein thrombosis) and lungs (pulmonary embolism) have been reported with EVISTA. Women who have or have had blood clots in the legs, lungs, or eyes should not take EVISTA. Women who have had a heart attack or are at risk for a heart attack may have an increased risk of dying from stroke when taking EVISTA. The most common side effects of EVISTA are hot flashes, leg cramps, swelling of the feet, ankles, and legs, flu syndrome, joint pain, and sweating. Hot flashes are more common during the first 6 months after starting treatment." These are not all the side effects of EVISTA.

Source: U.S. Food and Drug Administration (2007). Evista Medication Guide, ID: Eli Lilly and Company.

Teriparatide (Forteo) is typically prescribed for more severe osteoporosis and for individuals who have already had osteoporotic fractures. The following is the list of its side effects found on the FDA website:

"Decrease in blood pressure when you change positions. Some people feel dizzy, get a fast heartbeat, or feel faint right after the first few doses. This usually happens within 4 hours of taking FORTEO and goes away within a few hours. For the first few doses, take your injections of FORTEO in a place where you can sit or lie down right away if you get these symptoms. If your symptoms get worse or do not go away, stop taking FORTEO and call your healthcare provider. Increased calcium in blood. Tell your healthcare provider if you have nausea, vomiting, constipation, low energy, or muscle weakness. These may be signs there is too much calcium in your blood."
Common side effects of FORTEO include:

- nausea
- joint aches
- pain

"Your healthcare provider may take samples of blood and urine during treatment to check your response to FORTEO. Also, your healthcare provider may ask you to have follow-up

tests of bone mineral density. Tell your healthcare provider if you have any side effect that bothers you or that does not go away."
Source: U.S. Food and Drug Administration (2002). Forteo Medication Guide, ID: Eli Lilly and Company

Myths about Osteoporosis

"Osteoporosis is just a natural part of aging."

Osteoporosis and aging have a correlation relationship, not a causation relationship. Lifestyle changes, caused by decreasing mechanical loading on the body, force prevalence of this disease in the aging populations, but the disease is not caused by aging in itself. This is one of the most common misconceptions about osteoporosis: That we are all doomed to futures of being hunched over or suffering from broken hips. Osteoporosis is a degradation in bone density, and it can be significantly affected by high-impact levels of axial mechanical loading.

"I take calcium so I don't have to worry about osteoporosis."

There are actually 17 nutrients that are critical for bone health, and calcium is just one of them. However, the misconception of calcium being the answer to the osteoporosis problem has led many to take calcium dietary supplements in excess, which not only does not solve the bone health problem but creates other adverse health conditions such as increased risk of kidney stones (Curhan, et al., 1997).

Even when the body is given all of the proper nutrients for bone health, these are just building blocks. The function of bone tissue increasing in mass or gaining in density is using these building blocks only as an adaptive response to a stimulus. So without the stimulus for the adaptive response, the body cannot use these building blocks. The function of bone mass density generation involves axial bone loading. Once intense loading happens, the bone mass genesis (osteoblast) begin to retain minerals, and the bone mass becomes more dense.

"I exercise, so I don't have to worry about osteoporosis."

The mechanics of running include a heel strike impact, resulting in three to four times as much force as the body weight of the individual, depending on speed (Heinonen, et al., 1996). For this reason, more injuries result from running or impact-type fitness activity than non-weight bearing exercise. This has forced many physicians to encourage low-impact or non-weight bearing exercise (such as cycling) for older individuals (Hopkins, et al., 1990, Robinson, et al., 1998, Rector, et al., 2008) in order to prevent osteoporosis. In 2008 a study was published comparing bone health in adult male recreational athletes, aged 20 to 59, belonging to two groups, one group being cyclists (non-weight bearing exercisers), the other group being runners, (weight-bearing exercisers), whose impact loads are beyond their body weight. Of the cyclists 63%had osteopenia of the spine or hip (determined by DXA scans), compared with only 19% in the running group. "Cyclists were 7 times more likely to have osteopenia of the spine than runners, controlling for age, body weight, and bone-loading history. Based on the results of this study, current bone loading is an important determinant of whole-body and lumbar spine bone mass density. Therefore, bone-loading activity should be sustained during adulthood to maintain bone mass." (Rector, et al., 2008)

"I will only be concerned with this disease after I break a bone, which isn't that big of a deal."

Individuals with osteoporosis can be asymptomatic, with diagnosis of osteoporosis only after a fracture. Obviously this is not desirable or logical. Cooper, et al. reported that individuals over the age of 50 who break the hip or femur head have a higher mortality in the year following their fracture resulting from their immobility during the recovery (1993). In 1993 the Mayo Clinic did a retrospective analysis of osteoporotic vertebral fracture patients. At five years post-diagnosis of the fracture, the survival rate was 61%. "Clinically diagnosed vertebral fractures are rarely fatal, and the reduced survival seen subsequently could relate to comorbid conditions." (Cooper, et al., 1993) This means the presence of other diseases or disorders can contribute to the higher death rate, and the inability to move or fully use lung capacity, raise heart rate, or use nutrients properly compounds risk.

"One of my parents had Osteoporosis, I suppose I am going to have it also."

There are genetic indicators for this disease. However as the disease involves a lack of axial loading being imposed on the body, both the onset and degree of the disease can be delayed. Genetic predisposition is one contributing factor to the disease. Others include the following (Ralston, 2005):

- Certain kidney diseases
- Vitamin D deficiency
- Some hormonal diseases, such as some thyroid disorders
- Cushing's syndrome
- Treatment with steroids for certain medical conditions
- Certain types of cancer

"I am male, and this is a disease that affects females; therefore, I have nothing to worry about."

Though it is more prevalent in women, men can certainly be affected by osteoporosis. The International Osteoporosis Foundation estimates that, in the United States, almost two million men have osteoporosis and another three million are at risk (IOF, 2010). No different from women, osteoporotic men suffer from osteoporotic fractures in hips, spine, wrists, and other bones.

"I will look into osteoporosis when I am older; I am too young to worry about it now."

Looking at bone mass is not simple. Bone mass increases or decreases depend on the levels of proper stimulus. Commonly, younger individuals receive more axial loading of the bone mass, therefore achieving a higher level of bone mass density. When the individual stops inducing high-impact level loads, the result is degradation of bone mass, but this process can take years. Individuals who ignore the lack of axial mechanical loading being placed on the skeletal system can begin degradation of bone mass density. Ultimately, when the individual does finally address the issue, bone mass is already low, and attempting to load the body via conventional exercise modalities becomes more difficult and has an elevated chance of fracture.

More importantly, up to 90% of bone mass is created during childhood and adolescence. A specific example would be the bone mass density differences in both the lumbar spine and femoral neck. During puberty the mass density of bone tissue can increase from four to six times in both males and females. This is the period when both the size and density of the skeleton grows. This phenomenon, called "peak bone mass," can continue to develop up to the age of thirty. Typically, bone mass begins to slowly decline, then accelerates at the onset of menopause for women. Considering that most of the bone mass individuals will have in their lives develops before the age of thirty, it would make sense to have individuals focus on maximal bone loading from adolescence on. The greater the bone mass is at the time of peak bone mass, the higher the bone mass will be in later decades of life.

CHAPTER 6

CONVENTIONAL TRAINING

METHODS AND LIMITATIONS

Conventional resistance training is effective for almost all adult populations, ranging from athlete to the deconditioned, from those 18 years of age to their final years. The protocols and techniques used for different athletic skills and ages depend on the conditioning level and interest of the individual. The following studies and observations about conventional resistance training illustrate some limitations in relation to myofibril hypertrophy and bone mass density development as applied to these populations:

Resistance Training —Not High Enough Loads to be Effective

While traditional resistance training has been demonstrated to positively affect muscle hypertrophy, the loads required to increase myofibril hypertrophy are difficult if not impossible to achieve with current technology. Petrella, (2008), in the *Journal of American Physiology* analyzed myofibril development in a test group and made the observation that, out of 66 subjects they selected, 17 had either no or nominal myofibril response to a conventional resistance training protocol. Intensity of stimulus is directly related to adaptive responses in the human body.

Loading, Multiples of Bodyweight

The observation has been made that loading that is affiliated with conventional resistance training is not of the level required to have more than a nominal effect on the osteoblastic function of bone mass, pointed out in the Journal of Bone and Mineral. Researchers Forwood and Burr (1993) in their study titled, "Physical activity and bone mass: exercises in futility?" state that with "moderate intensity exercise" only modest bone mass density changes can occur. Marcus (1996), a Stanford Endocrinology researcher, points out that most studies that have looked at bone mass development through exercise have focused on resistance training and running as methods of stimulation. Marcus points out that these activities show only modest change. He further points out that Heinonen et al. (1996) used high-impact exercise in an 18-month period and saw significant gains in the test group. The observations of the levels of loading are most profound:

> "Unexpectedly high BMD values in women gymnasts are intriguing in this regard, since gymnastic activity produces enormous skeletal impacts (about 18 body weights with each dismount from parallel bars) with few loading cycles. Using fairly high-impact activity, Heinonen et al. found BMD gains of 1·4-3·7% by 18 months. Although significant, these increases do not substantially exceed those reported for other forms of endurance or resistance activity, perhaps because the training impacts actually achieved were not very large. The authors calculate their jump-training to have induced peak forces below 6 body weights, little more than the 3–4 body-weight forces associated with jogging. To fully

exploit the skeletal potential of impact loading might therefore require activities so rigorous that safety would be jeopardized. The Heinonen paper offers new information about human skeletal response." (p. 1327)

Additional observations in impact level loading have been made, all showing similar results, but with a caveat of risk in use. (Robinson, et al. 1995, Friedlander, et al. 1995, Fuches, Baure, and Snow, 2001)

Biomechanical Inefficacy

With conventional resistance training, individuals experience momentary muscular failure in less than optimal ranges of motion. Such a small number of myofibrils within the sarcomere structures are engaged in this weak range of motion that the ultimate stimulus to the CNS lacks appropriate intensity. Since the most intense stimulus will yield an adaptive or comparatively larger adaptive response, this activity will not produce a myofibril adaptation effectively. Individuals engaging in conventional resistance training should not be discouraged, as they are still stimulating sarcoplasmic hypertrophy, along with creating a circulatory benefit.

Benefits of High-Impact Training May Not Outweigh the Risks

Heinonen (1996) focused on high-impact exercise on lower limb bone mass density with postmenopausal women. Heinonen's hypothesis was that magnitudes of force were thought to be essential for maximizing skeletal adaptive response. The initial test group consisted of 242 women, with a reduced study sample size of 98. The significant reduction in sample size was due to the protocol requirements that included regular exercise more than twice a week, as well as having no chronic disease that might limit training or testing. Subjects were then randomly assigned into equal training and control groups. Of the training group only 39 completed the 18-week high-impact program because of aggravation to previous musculoskeletal problems, pregnancy, accidental back injury, lower limb overuse injury, and other factors. Though the conclusion of the research had positive outcomes in improving skeletal integrity and increasing bone mass density, the benefits were only seen in a small fraction of the initial sample pool.

An article published in *Osteoporosis International* by Bassey and Ramsdale, (1984) compared low-impact and high-impact exercise. After six months of training, the low-impact group had no statistically significant gain in bone mass. The high-impact group showed an increase of 3.4% in femoral bone density. The *Journal of Orthopaedic Trauma* stated "Significant and possibly irreversible articular cartilage damage occurs after a single high-energy impact load" (Borrelli, et al., 1997). This presents a question: Is the actual impact on bone tissue the stimulus that leads to the creation of bone mass density, or is it the load that is used, up to multiples of the individual's body weight, that stimulates bone mass density creation? This is important because mechanical loading of multiples of bodyweight without impact would lead to a safer method of bone loading.

Verhoshanski (1968) suggested that, due to danger of injury, it would be ill-advised to allow a beginning athlete to engage in jump training as such high-impact activity should only be used with individuals of a "high level of sports mastery." Blattner and Nobel (1977) also stated that a disadvantage of jump or high-impact training is the potential of injury.

Loading Origin Limitation

The definition of concentric contraction is one in which the muscle shortens through a range of motion. While conventional fitness/exercise equipment involves imposing loading on the body, the physical reality of conventional full-range exercise will inherently limit an individual in his or her ability to use higher (or the highest possible) loads. When an individual picks up a free weight, such as a barbell, he or she is limited by the capacity to hold, balance, and manage the weight as it moves through the range of the exercise.

During conventional exercise, an individual goes to momentary muscular failure in a full range of motion departing from the optimal biomechanical range. This is the normal protocol of conventional exercise, but by definition this range of motion involves less engagement of the muscle cells, also referred to as myofibril engagement, and a decreased degree of possible force output. When going to momentary muscular failure in this weaker range of motion, the individual is also in the exercise commonly associated with muscular and joint injury. The individual gives a maximal effort at a joint angle where the least amount of force production is possible.

The definition of eccentric contraction is one in which the muscle elongates through the motion because the action potential is less than the force or load being applied to it. An example of this would be seen in an individual's ability to lower a given weight or load but not the ability to be able to actually lift or raise that load.

This type of eccentric contraction occurs after momentary muscular failure takes place. An individual exerciser goes to momentary muscular failure but then must do something with the load. Lowering this load facilitates opportunity for injury. In 1990 the Department of Physical Education at the University of Georgia compiled exercise data that showed that, following eccentric contractions, damage in myofibrillar units within sarcomeres appears. (Armstrong, 1990) When looking at the different types of muscular development/hypertrophy, the opportunity for sarcoplasmic growth stimulation exists in this type of contraction.

A Better Way to Achieve Impact Level Loading is Needed

In an effort to achieve loading of the body, many individuals will select weights in conventional training modalities that are beyond what should be considered as safe. In an article featured in *The New York Times*, data was presented showing that from 1992 to 2007 nearly one million Americans were treated in hospital emergency rooms as a result of injury from conventional resistance training exercise injuries. The article made note that women predominantly injured their feet and legs and also had a greater portion of fractures, while men had more injuries of the hands and trunk, as well as sprains. Most interesting was the fact that the majority of injury occurred when individuals dropped weights on themselves, thereby crushing a body part between two weights or hitting themselves with the equipment (Bakalar, 2010).

CHAPTER 7

NEW TECHNOLOGY TO

EFFECTIVELY DEAL WITH THE

LIMITATIONS

To build both myofibril muscular development, and bone mass density, loads must be applied to the body that approach the loading levels of impact. Current resistance technology is limited in the level of loading that can be safely applied to the human body. A new-patented technology has been introduced that allows for significantly greater loading of both muscular and bone tissue. Two key principles were applied to accomplish the objective:

1. **Isolating Optimal Biomechanical Ranges:** The device chassis allows for both gross and fine anatomical adjustments allowing optimal biomechanical positioning repeatable from one osteogenic exposure session to the next. Isolating this range of motion allows for stimulus to the musculoskeletal system that meets the requirement of loading the body at the levels provided by high-impact training in activity.

2. Loading Origin: Unlike conventional resistance training equipment, the origin of the loading event is the individual using the device. The load is self-induced, meaning the only load an individual would be imposing on his or her musculoskeletal system would be voluntarily created by muscular contraction in the optimal biomechanical position. This is unlike any conventional exercise where load is imposed on an individual through the act of holding a weight and moving it through space or managing the movement of a load via a cable apparatus (common in conventional resistance facilities).

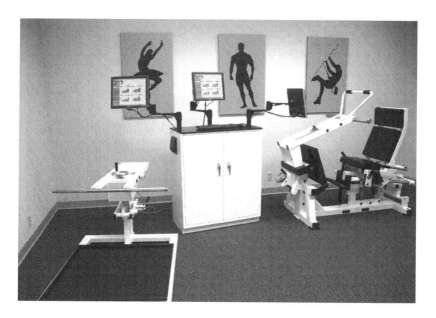

Figure 7-1, The original bioDensity device prototype

Osteogenic Loading - bioDensity

In 2005, the bioDensity device was first prototyped, shown above. This device was created to be both a safe and nonintimidating tool to induce impact-level loading of the neuro-musculoskeletal system in optimal biomechanical ranges of motion. Along with hardware, software was required to manage these osteogenic loading events. This software needed to give the individual using the device both useful and encouraging information, as well as provide the medical professional who is examining the results with loading and adaptation information. The following were the requirements of the software system:

1. Software for the User Experience - The software developed to run the device would allow for individual user accounts that would track and analyze the performance of an individual user, as well as encourage the user through each load exposure by displaying previous performances for motivation and maintain safety through the exposure. An example of the performance report is shown below (User: male, 35):

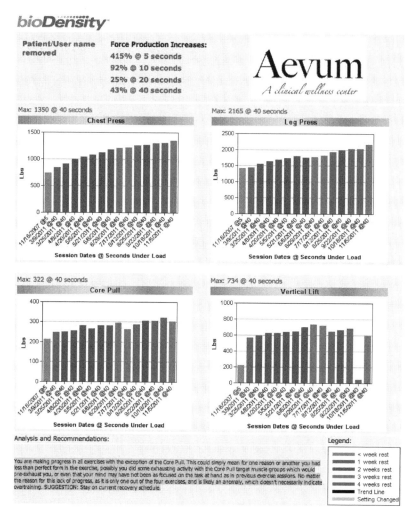

Figure 7-2, bioDensity Performance Report

2. Monitoring Adaptation - A patented algorithm allows for optimizing repeat osteogenic exposures.

3. Network Design - The software solution is managed through a network service, also known as an application

service provider function (ASP), in order to simplify operations of each treatment location to make the experience consistent from one location to the next. This means managing the data would not be the burden of a location operator; rather everything would be managed from a centralized server. All data collected by the server would be used in further analysis for all subsequent sessions.

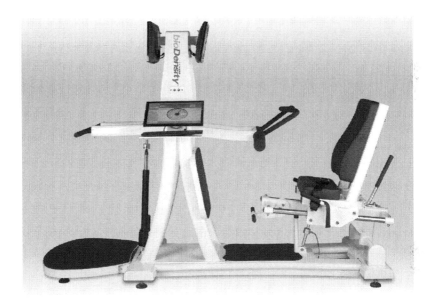

Figure 7-3, The more compact/current bioDensity model

Osteoporosis and the bioDensity Device

Research has shown that exercise that involves high impact can reverse bone loss and add bone mineral density where previously it was lost, but with this osteogenic loading technology, the practice and practicality of impact-level loading is possible. This simple intervention increases strength, power, balance, and coordinative abilities. Osteogenic loading on bioDensity may offer relief from crippling conditions related to loss of bone mineral density, osteopenia, and osteoporosis.

Osteoporosis is an illness that threatens millions. While men and women suffer from osteoporosis, the majority of sufferers in the U.S. are women, comprising 80% of the diagnosed cases. One woman in two and one man in four will break a bone due to osteoporosis. With a net loss of bone matrix, individuals are more vulnerable to fracture: every 10% of bone loss results in a redoubling of fracture risk. Prevention is the key, as frail bones can lead to debilitating health after a fracture. Maintaining strong bones is considered an important anti-aging intervention (Mundy, 1999).

Can osteoporosis be prevented? Research says yes, by using exercise, a balanced diet, the avoidance of heavy drinking and smoking, and medical interventions. The factors people have the most control over are the factors that will help prevent osteoporosis. Many are not able to exercise safely: walking outside may cause falls, and many elderly people would rather not visit health clubs or gyms. Osteogenic loading with bioDensity offers a safe, gentle, achievable means to exercise for millions of at-risk people.

Prevention of osteoporosis with bioDensity use may avoid the potentially harmful side effects of medical interventions, such as pharmaceuticals. The use of the device is pleasant, accessible, easy to do, takes little time, and can provide measurable improvements in the health of our aging population. It has served as an important tool for helping to slow down the degenerative process of the entire human body.

Isolating Optimal Biomechanical Ranges

Achieving both maximum myofibril engagement and skeletal mechanical leverage is required for an optimal biomechanical osteogenic exposure. Though it is simple enough just to look at maximum myofibril engagement, ignoring skeletal mechanical leverage would abandon chances of the highest loads possible. For this reason multi-joint movements were chosen as a starting point for the chassis of the device to be developed. Four optimal biomechanical positions were chosen. The selection of multi-joint motion has been favored in sports performance training for many decades because the positions mimic natural motion. As these motions in sports performance training were not carried out with limitations on range of motion, benefits of myofibril engagement or skeletal mechanical leverage were not relevant.

For example, a common exercise apparatus found in a health club is a quadricep extension. When watching an individual perform this conventional exercise, in looking at the involvement of the quadricep muscles (front thigh muscles), it is obvious that tremendous involvement of the quadricep is required. Sports performance trainers, however, will not readily select this exercise for athletes. They instead prefer squatting or leg-press type actions. From a biomechanical standpoint this motion or action is what the body does in a natural situation. In other words,, standing up from the floor or even running involve the glutes, quadriceps, hamstrings, and calves (a majority of muscles in the lower legs) as they all work together. So the CNS will respond to a stimulus of natural motion and not necessarily to isolation-type exercise, such as the quadricep extension exercise apparatus.

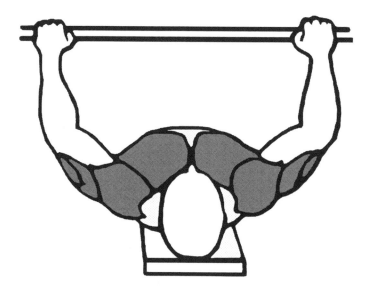

Figure 7-5, The position of optimal biomechanics

Each session on the bioDensity device requires monitoring by a technician. From a casual user standpoint, one session of four load exposures—where the entire time under tension is only 20 seconds— does not leave enough time for the user to remember how to use the software. Also, in the load exposure sessions, users are loading the body with between hundreds and, at times, upwards of 4000 pounds. In this situation care must be taken to make sure the protocols are followed, and each session is safe for the user. The software has been developed to dis-incentivize improper behaviors, such as rapid loading, or exploding into a load exposure. Requiring a technician is not necessarily cumbersome for a medical facility that employs this technology since for each individual, though under tension for only a matter of seconds, the entire session can take approximately 5 minutes.

Osteogenic Loading Counteracts Deconditioning

The aging process is often affiliated with loss of strength, decreased bone density, lower ability to deliver oxygen to tissues, atrophy in the cardiovascular muscles, hormone changes, inability to product force, and loss of efficiency. The use of osteogenic loading helps avoid these adverse conditions.

Osteogenic loading is an appropriate, versatile, and safe modality for maintaining muscle activation in the arms and legs, as well as activating motoneurons, a critical link to the body's sensitivity to balance (Hebb, 1949, Taube, 2011). Most important, for populations who cannot engage in conventional exercise or resistance training, there is an indication that safe, self-controlled loading using the bioDensity device can counteract the effects of bed rest, sedentary lifestyle, and bone loss.

Power

The use of osteogenic loading enhances power. Power is also called "speed strength," the ability of an individual to create a loading event, with rapid creation of force being the primary objective. Speed strength is vital during a great many functional demands and movements such as sport, play, active daily living, and response to emergencies, such as preventing a fall or dodging an obstacle. Power is the body's preferred method of generating force; when you lift a heavy object, speed assists in the lift. Power and speed strength exercise are important in improving intramuscular coordination, which is the ability to recruit a high threshold of motor units to perform a certain motion. In conventional training, prior to power training, athletes needed a foundation of absolute strength, endurance, and agility.

With the use of osteogenic loading, power and speed are developed for three reasons:

1. Increase occurs in contractile tissue, myofibril hypertrophy.

2. More muscle tissue is recruited with power movements via potentiation.

3. Bone tissue is reinforced, thereby increasing loading comfort.

Individuals engaging in conventional fitness programs would normally see power as an advanced training goal in conventional training environments' however, with the bioDensity device, all users experience improved power and force production. To train for power, the following factors are required to generate force: stabilization, strength, skill, and speed. The osteogenic loading stimulation prepares the body for all aspects of power simultaneously and generates greater neuromuscular recruitment in the body.

Transferability

The strength in the myofibril development provided by this technology transfers to all ranges of motion. Considering the fact that there is use of only a limited range of motion in bioDensity, this brings up many questions. The simple answer is that, as the stimulus is engaged in the optimal biomechanical range of motion, by definition all-potential myofibrils are both involved, and stimulated. Therefore, even with low levels of myofibril involvement in the weaker ranges of motion, realize increases in strength. Barak, Ayalon, and Dvir (2004) demonstrated that limited range of motion resistance training is able to translate into full-range strength gains. Johnston (2005) concluded, "no evidence exists to the effect that muscle development is contingent on full range exercise." Mookerjee, and Ratamess (1999) observed strength gains through the entire range of motion when isolating the optimal biomechanical position.

Conclusion

The level of axial mechanical loading that osteogenic loading provides is a proven resource for maintaining and improving bone density, strength, circulation, power, fat loss, coordination, and overall improved wellness. It is a viable and safe option for those people who are unwilling or unable to perform high-impact training or heavy conventional resistance training exercises and for at-risk populations. Prevention is the best strategy for avoiding the risks of osteoporosis. Regular use of the bioDensity device offers many people an accessible and viable solution for rebuilding bone and being trained to avoid falls.

The bioDensity stimulus is not designed to replace any type of exercise or therapy. The device is designed to facilitate the type of stimulus that is unrealistic to attain in most athletic or exercise endeavor. The bioDensity device will not be the only of its kind. This is a new modality of therapy that individuals will be able to realize the benefits of. The larger implication of this technology is safely increasing the loads on the body that will have positive outcomes on bone density, balance, metabolism, rehabilitation, and high- performance athletics. Individuals of all ages and all levels of physical fitness—from those deconditioned to professional/high-performance athletes - will be able to safely gain a higher power-to-weight ratio and a stronger skeletal structure.

CHAPTER 8

HISTORY OF

BIODENSITY/OSTEOGENIC

LOADING DEVELOPMENT, USERS,

AND ACCURACY

Wolff's Law:

"As a consequence of primary shape variations and continuous loading, or even due to loading alone, bone changes its inner architecture according to mathematical rules and, as a secondary effect and, governed by the same mathematical rules, also changes its shape."
- Julius Wolff, 1892

A Retrospective Analysis

Originating from the observation of Wolff's law, a retrospective analysis was conducted based on human activities and exercise at California State University Sacramento in 1997. The initial task was defining specific adaptations from activities individuals could engage in through adulthood to enhance their health and quality of life. The individual areas needing improvement to enhance the quality of life for aging individuals were as follows:

1. Bone density
2. Muscular strength
3. Posture
4. Balance

All of these areas of wellness degrade with age. Therefore, the discovery of a process that could slow age-related degradation or even reverse that degradation would be beneficial. In this retrospective paper, focus was placed on the decades of life where the areas of wellness listed above are improving instead of degrading. Wolff's law, simply stated, says that mechanical loading of bone tissue will create an adaptive response that increases the density of bone tissue. Though this has been understood by modern medicine for more than 100 years, diminishing bone mass density, (osteoporosis) continues to affect millions of people. Research published a year before the retrospective showed that impact delivers mechanical loading that is up to multiples of body weight, and this level of loading is required for the creation and maintenance of bone mass density (Marcus, 1986). More recently in "Bone Health and Osteoporosis: A Report of the Surgeon General" (2004) the U.S. Surgeon General states that activities that "involve impact are most useful for increasing or maintaining bone mass."

As the levels of mechanical loading, needed for the adaptive response in bone mass are far higher than can be handled safely with conventional therapy (Borrelli, et al., 1997, Slemenda, et al., 1991, Whalen, et al., 1988), the conclusion of the retrospective was that a device was needed that allowed for mechanical loading that was of levels equivalent to that of impact, and with minimized risk of injury.

To create axial mechanical loading effects on the body that are multiples of an individual's body weight and are available to a broad population, a new and unique device would have to be designed. There were three engineering concepts employed to make this innovation possible:

1. This device would have to isolate the optimal biomechanical positions an individual would naturally assume for absorbing impact in the safest way.

2. This device would have to allow for self-created loading, so that the CNS regulates the limitations of the individual. This provides a low risk of injury.

3. This device would have to provide computerized biofeedback, so the individual would be able to see the loading event in real time.

Osteogenic Loading – bioDensity, the First Application, and First Test Users

In 2005 the term *osteogenic loading* was reported as the application of the highest possible loads in optimal positions managed via computer device and commercially branded as bioDensity.

Beta testing on the first generation of the bioDensity device began in January 2005 and continued until January 2009. During this time 400 individuals were exposed to a total of 40,000 osteogenic loading sessions of one per week or one bi-weekly, depending on algorithm-generated suggestion. Of the initial beta subjects, a sub set of eight individuals were pre-screened with DXA scans for evaluation of bone density. The subjects were exposed to osteogenic loading on the bioDensity device over a period of 36 months, averaging one use every other week. The group consisted of 7 females and

1 male, mean age 67.2 +/-9.4 years. All eight individuals were diagnosed with osteopenia or osteoporosis. Over the period of osteogenic loading use, there were no injuries to any of the subject group, and all individuals completed the entire loading protocol. At the completion of the period, each of the subjects was exposed to a second DXA scan under the same conditions as the first scan. All subjects showed positive outcomes.

As each DXA scan used different anatomical locations and varying DXA scanning machines, the results were reported differently:

Subject 1: 86 year old female. Bone mass density of the spine increased by 2.8% from the previous exam. Hip bone mass density increased 1.1% from the previous exam. The subject was taking medication to prevent bone mass loss.

Subject 2: 59 year old female. Increase in bone mass density of the spine of 6%. This subject was not taking medication for bone mass loss and was doing no other heavy loading of the musculoskeletal system.

Subject 3: 71 year old female. Bone mass density of the lumbar spine increased by 5% from the previous exam. Femoral bone mass density increased 1% from the previous exam. This subject was not taking medication for bone mass loss and described her other physical activity as "dancing and walking."

Subject 4: 70 year old male. This subject had not had a DXA scan for six years. The second DXA scan was administered 36 months after beginning osteogenic loading. From the age of 64 to 70 patient has not had significant bone mass loss, therefore, was not at higher risk of fracture. The subject took no medication for bone mass loss and described his other activities as "mild bicycling."

Subject 5: 62 year old female. Bone mass density of the lumbar spine increased by 3.4% from the previous exam. The subject took no medication for bone mass loss and described her other physical activity as "aerobics 3 to 4 times a week."

Subject 6: 59 year old female. Bone mass density of the spine increased by 6% from the previous exam. Hip bone mass density had no significant change from the previous exam. The subject took no medication for bone mass loss and described her other physical activity as "aerobics 3 to 4 times a week."

Subject 7: 61 year old female. Bone mass density of the lumbar spine increased, test results show .954 gm/cm² up from .821 gm/cm² a T Score of -0.8 a classification of normal, up from -2.1 which is a classification of osteopenia. This subject took no medication for bone mass loss and described her other physical activity as "dance frequently, ride bike and hike."

Subject 8: 79 year old female. Improvements from a diagnosis of osteoporosis to a diagnosis of osteopenia. Bone mass density of the lumbar spine increased. Test results show a T Score of -2.1, up from -3.1. There were hip density improvements as well, with a T Score of -1.6, up from -1.8. This subject took no medication to prevent bone mass loss and described her other physical activity as "moderate activity."

The detailed case reports are in Chapter 18.

Over the four-year period, 400 individuals volunteered for the osteogenic loading protocol of one time per week with the bioDensity device. After four years of testing some accomplishments it made are as following:

1. 40,000 load exposure sessions had been recorded with the bioDensity machine.

2. An average age of 52 years was characteristic of the group of 400 test subjects.

3. No recorded injuries occurred in any of the 40,000 osteogenic loading sessions.

Currently there are over 400,000 osteogenic loading sessions in the database with still no recorded injuries.

Accuracy

The bioDensity device was conceived to provide highly accurate weekly performance reports. Traditional fitness equipment systems are not necessarily known for being accurate or repeatable. Load cells with high accuracy were chosen as the device of measurement to be incorporated into the bioDensity device. They also have low nonlinearity occurrence (0.15%), meaning the reading of increases and decreases in load have low variance.

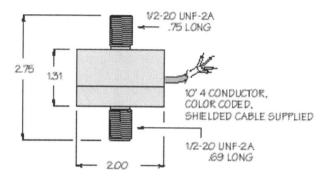

Figure 8-1, An Illustration of the type of load cells used in the bioDensity device

Dead weights and transfer standards and all measurement equipment used to calibrate the load cells are certified on a regular schedule. The procedure for calibration includes four load points, which are recorded from zero to full scale increasing and decreasing, with the errors documented as linearity and hysteresis as percent of full scale. This procedure is repeated and the difference between runs documented for repeatability error as percent of full scale. Finally, with the load cell sensor at zero (NO LOAD) position, a precision wire-wound resistor is placed across the power lead and signal lead, producing a millivolt output. The calibration certificate will reflect the resistor value and millivolt output, along with calculated percent of full scale.

The bioDensity Networked System Accuracy Requirements:

Because the bioDensity™ system utilizes its own Application Service Provider (ASP) function residing in a central server connected to each bioDensity™ system, the ASP function allows all information and support software to reside on a host system using a thin-client hardware configuration. This design provides owners and users with data that is updated instantly and accessible wherever the session takes place. The nature of the bioDensity™ system assures that movements are measured with accuracy and consistency, irrespective of the specific bioDensity™ unit being used. This latter point allows any user worldwide to receive accurate measurement on any bioDensity machine, with the last session data displayed. The user can also engage in the next exercise with the same accuracy and repeatability as though the user was on the machine that he or she normally uses.

CHAPTER 9

ADAPTIVE RESPONSE:

NEURAL POTENTIATION

The osteogenic loading stimulation of the neuro-musculoskeletal system provides a CNS adaptive response immediately upon use. Bhem (2004) illustrated an increase in short-term explosive force neural potentiation with short-duration and high resistance maximal voluntary contractions. This type of stimulation can be easily facilitated with osteogenic loading since the nature of maximal myofibril engagement provides high levels of fiber recruitment. Thus, the individual engages the action potential to the greatest degree.

Increased neural activity (H-reflex amplitudes) shows the evidence of a post-contraction explosive force neural potentiation, determined by Gullich and Schmidtbleicher's (1996) and Aagaard, et al, (2002). This amplification can exist 10 minutes following the contraction (Trimble and Harp, 1998). This effect, known as Post-Activation Potential (PAP), means that the body is encouraged to perform at a greater level and has more force-generating capacity.

Athletic Implications

Elastic Equivalent Training is a method of physical training used by high-performance athletes that partners strength exercise with power/explosiveness exercise, in that order. The neural potentiation goal is to activate the CNS to the highest degree with the strength exercise, then immediately move to the power/explosive movement so that the second movement is performed with a greater level of CNS activity. This provides both better performance and better stimulus for further development. The practice of using bioDensity to prime an athlete for an explosive event would be taking the already popular practice of Elastic Equivalent Training to the highest degree. Positive effect can also be seen in stability endurance. By activating the H-reflex amplitudes and the maximal levels of fiber recruitment with bioDensity, an athlete can increase stability in functional positions while training within this same window. When training an athlete, the use of bioDensity should be to amplify the other aspects of training.

Aging Population Implications

Though Elastic Equivalent Training as described above may be slightly impractical for individuals past the sixth or seventh decade of life, the principle may still apply. An individual can use the bioDensity device, then immediately move to an activity that he or she is comfortable with, but the most explosive that he or she would naturally encounter. For elderly individuals, even activities like repeatedly getting out of a chair, then sitting down again could fall into this category. Here the element of stability endurance comes into play as well. Almost as important as the physiological changes that are made in the individual who is pairing bioDensity and chair training is the level of confidence this action builds.

Long-Term Potentiation and Neural Network Implications

"What fires together, wires together," (Hebb, 1949), meaning when one engages muscular cells in action, the cells working together even more effectively over time. Motor learning, also called long-term potentiation, begin this way, and as the individual repeats and speeds the action, greater neural adaptive response takes place. Taube (2011) suggests through review of studies on maximal voluntary contractions not only shows the neural potentiation change in immediate twitch force, but slow sustained maximal voluntary contractions share similarities to building long-term potentiation. The more force an individual produces repeatedly over time in an action, the greater the nervous system involvement with future action. Use of the bioDensity device provides individuals the opportunity for these maximal voluntary contractions, which then can enhance the functioning of the nervous system.

Enhanced Reflex Action

Proprioception is the subconscious connection of the CNS to engage skeletal muscular tissue when needed. The proprioceptors are nervous system receptors located throughout joints, muscles, and tendons. They relay information through both the conscious (action potential for an intended movement) and subconscious (reflexive, e.g. catching one's self in the process of falling and repositioning to maintain balance) parts of the CNS to initiate conscious action. When an individual increases the force production in an exercise, proprioception enables greater cross sectional muscular fiber recruitment. This is the first adaptive response.

CHAPTER 10

ADAPTIVE RESPONSE:

MYOFIBRIL DEVELOPMENT

Optimal Biomechanics

McKenzie & Gandevia (1987) analyzed muscular performance at the shortest possible lengths and the enhanced endurance of maximal voluntary contractions. A follow-up to the study in the next year examined the ability to voluntarily engage muscular tissue at the fixed positions (Gandevia & McKenzie, 1988). Though the purpose was not necessarily to identify optimal biomechanical ranges of motion, the researchers examined the concept that the shortest possible position, when the muscle is completely engaged, would produce the greatest force output. The results showed that, though complete motor neuron activation was possible in a muscle's shortest possible position (complete contraction at the end of joint movement), the force production in that fixed position declined by 21 to 49%. The control contractions were performed short of the end of potential joint movement. The researchers concluded from the data that complete motor neuron engagement and the highest possible force production are possible in this limited range of motion. Previous studies involving isometric exercise looked at varying static positions but rarely looking at mechanically positioning the body so that target muscles were in the shortest possible position for increased loading. Identifying the position of optimal biomechanics—or, stated differently, the position in which an individual can create the greatest amount of force— is key in delivering the most powerful or intense stimulus to the target muscular tissue.

Observations over many years in both sports training and general exercise have shown that best adaptive responses in the human body occur with the most intense stimulus (Tsuzuku, et al., 2001, Fiatrone, et al., 1990). However, the intensity of the stimulus is often confused with the maximal effort. From a CNS perspective, effort, and stimulation have little in common. Having an individual use a given load or weight and exercise to the point of momentary muscular failure could be beneficial, depending on what the given load is and how is it applied. Many individuals do not adapt from the stimulus of standard exercise, mainly because they are unable to impose significant loading when in the optimal position of biomechanics. As stated above, this is the position where, in a given movement, the largest amount of force production is possible. By causing momentary muscular failure in this position, and only in this position, a much more intense stimulus is delivered to the target muscle tissue, thereby creating the potential for the greater adaptive response of myofibril development.

Applications of Optimal Biomechanics

The Olympic training group in the Soviet Union is credited with making the observation that isolating the optimal biomechanical range of motion for loading produces the greatest adaptive response. This is detailed by one of the architects of the Soviet Union's athletic success in the book *Science and Practice of Strength Training* (Zatsiorsky, 1995, p. 63). The Soviet athletes would participate in standard weight training activities and arrange their weight training equipment bars and machines so that the resistance was only placed on the athletes in the ranges that yielded maximal force production. This practice became commonly known as "block presses" and "box squats." Block presses entail placing wooden blocks on the chest of an individual while performing a standard bench press exercise. The individual un-racks the weight above, then lowers the bar only to where the bar touches the block, then repeats by moving the bar back upward in this short range of motion. This range is only 2 to 5 inches, but at close to full extension of the arms in the movement.

Box squats are a similar type of movement, involving a squat instead of a bench press. Individuals doing this exercise would un-rack the bar, then squat down in a very limited range of motion, staying close to full extension of the leg until sitting down on a wooden box built to a height specifically for them. Through staying in the optimal biomechanical range of motion during these exercises, the weights/loads they used were far higher than those the athletes would use in a full range of motion. After the fall of the Soviet Union, these principles made their way to the United States. Few strength and conditioning trainers applied these techniques, however, due to the increased danger as these higher weights/loads were used.

This type of training is often done through a conventional fitness apparatus, known in the powerlifting world as a "power rack." Instead of using blocks of wood on the chest, or building boxes specific to limiting the "sitting down" action of the squat exercise, the power rack is used to limit the range of motion of a given exercise. The same limited ranges of motion can be used in these power racks; however, they were not developed specifically for this purpose. Using the larger loads that are required for optimal biomechanical ranges of training, even in a power rack, does not reduce the risk of injury.

No direct explanation of why "block presses" and "box squats" would develop the highest levels of strength was offered by the Soviet athletic trainers. Wilson (1989) offered the idea, in the *International Journal of Sports Bio-mechanics*, that this limited, optimal biomechanical range of motion would decrease the neural inhibition in response to extreme loads. Subsequent research supports Wilson's conclusion that this adaptive response from the nervous system does indeed take place. However, the adaptive response in the mechanical cellular function is synergistic with the neural potentiation adaptation as well. An individual is both increasing the amount of contractile tissue, as well as being able to engage more tissue that is already there.

Mookerjee and Ratamass (1999) conducted a study in which subjects were tested to compare the results of exercizing a full range of motion bench press and a partial range of motion bench press. Mookerjee and Ratamass used a slightly larger range in their partial-range exercises, as opposed to training protocols the Soviet athletic trainers used. This range was determined by lowering the bar from a position of full extension down to a 90° angle in the elbow joint. The intent of the study was to train in a range of motion where "supra-maximal" loads would be used, meaning loads that exceed an individual's one-repetition maximum in a full range. The researchers used a point of reference from another study (Elliott, et al. 1989) that detailed the "sticking point" of a bench press movement, looking at both the biomechanical leverage of the bones involved and the potential engagement of the muscular tissue throughout the entire movement. Wilson, Elliott, and Kerr (1989) also identified the force profile characteristics of maximal loads in the bench press movement. They cited the 120° angle of the elbow joint in the action of the individual pushing the load straight away from his body to be the optimal biomechanical range of motion. Mookerjee and Ratamass found that their test group was able to impose far larger loads in their identified partial range of motion. In the comparison of one-repetition maximums, the test group was able to handle loads 4.78% greater than that of a full-range bench press motion. The researchers hypothesized that an individual who uses only the full range of motion might fail to engage the target muscles (triceps, deltoids, and pectorals) completely. It was suggested that imposing load in the optimal biomechanical range of motion produces maximal force and involves all target tissue. Thus, momentary muscular failure occurring in this optimal biomechanical range of motion will engage all myofibrils and stimulate the development of muscular myofibrils. The researchers concluded that their results showed that a significant increase in strength can occur with a single loading experience in the optimal biomechanical range of motion.

How, as Adults, do we Stimulate Myofibril Development?

Adults can stimulate myofibril development by imposing maximal loads in optimal biomechanical ranges of motion.

To fully understand the limitations of the different ranges of motion in a conventional exercise movement, we must look at an example. The following is an analysis of joint angles in a bench press exercise or any such exercise where both arms are used to push a load away from the body. A push-up exercise would be an example, as well as the use of many conventional types of exercise apparatus.

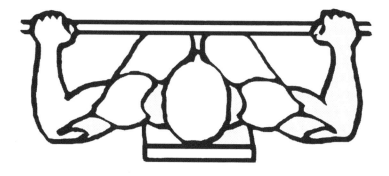

Figure 10-1, Stretched, non-optimal

Weaker Ranges of Motion

In figure 10-1 the individual has the load resting against his or her rib cage. Action potential begins from the CNS, then manifests as muscular contraction by the shortening of sarcomeres within the muscle cells. Each of the target muscles (triceps, deltoids, and pectorals) are in the most elongated position, therefore has the least myofibril engagement, so a minority of sarcomeres are engaged as the individual lifts the load off his or her rib cage. If figure 10-1 was depicting a push-up exercise instead of a bench press exercise, the image would be flipped upside down, and instead of grasping a bar the individual would have his or her hands on the floor, but the action in the movement described above would be identical.

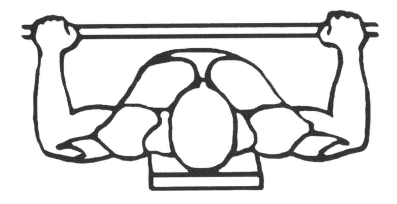

Figure 10-2, Partially contracted

In figure 10-2, the individual has moved the load so that the elbow is at a 90° angle. This is the position that the researchers Mookerjee and Ratamass used as the lower limit of their bench press experiment. This is defined as the "sticking point" of a bench press movement (Elliott, et al. 1989), meaning it is a range of motion where an exerciser will go to momentary muscular failure in a conventional full range of movement. Naming this joint angle the "sticking point" implies that it is the weakest point in a range of motion from a load production standpoint. More myofibril engagement occurs at this 90° angle than that depicted in figure 10-1; however mechanical leverage is poor.

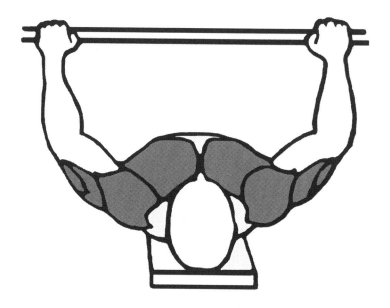

Figure 10-3, Optimal biomechanical range/Impact range

The Optimal Range of Motion

In figure 10-3 the optimal biomechanical range of motion is achieved. The elbow joint is at a 120° angle. This is not the shortest possible position for each target muscle; however, it is the shortest possible position that still allows for mechanical leverage in the skeletal structure of the arms and rib cage. This corresponds to the results the researchers McKenzie and Gandevia achieved by using electronmyography (a technology for evaluating and recording the electrical activity produced by skeletal muscles) to determine motor control function and force production as it relates to varying positions of joint angle. They found that greater force production is possible as muscles shorten. Going to momentary muscular failure in this position allows for loading that is beyond the one-repetition maximum of the individual and provides the stimulus required for myofibril muscular development.

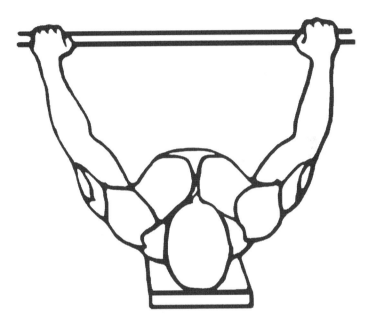

Figure 10-4, Fully extended range

Full Extention, Neuromuscular Limitation

In figure 10-4, the individual has departed from the optimal biomechanical range of motion and has lost mechanical leverage. The McKenzie and Gandevia study shows that, although each target muscle in the given movement is at its shortest possible position, electrical activity from the motor control function of the nervous system begins to limit the force the target muscles are able to produce.

Even in later stages of life, elderly individuals are able to increase muscle strength and cause adaptive responses, primarily via sarcoplasmic effect and possibly some myofibril effect, though the heavier loading required for myofibril effect is unlikely due to the risk of injury. In 1991, Charette, et al. conducted an experiment with 27 women (mean age 69+/-1year) to not only measure strength through a 12-week conventional resistance-training program, but also perform muscular biopsy (a surgically removed sample of the muscle) on each individual to look at changes in the muscular cross-sectional fiber. Biopsies were taken pre- and post-experiment from both the control group and the exercising group. The exercising subjects increased their strength values 28 to115% in all muscle groups, and there was no change in the control group. Muscular growth was seen primarily in type II fibers (20.1 +/- 6.8%, P = 0.02). This means that the volume of muscle cells/fibers increased; however, it is unlikely that this growth was myofibril (Charette, et al. 1991). These results show that aging individuals have little or no reason to disengage from exercise or fitness. However, the results of the Department of Health and Human Services analysis in 2000 showed that only 13 percent of individuals between ages 65 and 74 reported engaging in vigorous physical activity for 20 minutes 3 or more days per week, and only 6 percent of those 75 and older reported such exercise (U.S. HHS, 2000). No distinction was made between cardiovascular exercise activity and load-bearing exercise that is needed for either type of muscular development. In the 75-year plus category, the 6% statistic indicates how practical conventional resistance training is for the aging population.

The method described in isolating the optimal biomechanical position at the beginning of this chapter is also not practical for the general population. Having adult or aging adult members of the population use standard fitness/weight training apparatus to impose "supra-maximal" loading in an optimal biomechanical positions bears an excessive risk compared to the reward it could offer. Even though an individual exerciser is in a safer mechanical position, meaning staying away from the 90° angle as in the bench press example, the individual is still forced to impose a large load (relative to the individual) on him or herself. If the bar that is being held is gripped in an awkward fashion the individual must still manage the load he or she is holding, which may cause an injury.

Conclusion

The observations and bodies of research cited above point out a need for a solution that is applicable throughout an individual's lifetime. This solution must allow individuals to impose maximal loading in optimal biomechanical positions until the point of momentary muscular failure, and this must be achieved with a minimum risk of injury.

CHAPTER 11

ADAPTIVE RESPONSE: BONE

MASS DENSITY INCREASE

High-impact skeletal loading provides for positive adaptive response, as these loads approach or are multiples of the individual's bodyweight, and such loading forces osteoblastic action to retain minerals. It is the lack of skeletal loading that compromises the bone matrix over time, meaning loss of the ability to reinforce structure by retaining calcium and other key minerals. Endocrine limitations in the later decades of life (Sundar, et al., 2010) will also contribute to slow the loading of the ostoeblasts. Extreme examples of limitations in loading are pointed out by Whedon (1984) in *Calcified Tissue International*, in which he reported that even a short immobilization due to casts (for bone break or other reasons) and bed rest resulted in loss of bone matrix and calcium. If continued for many months, demineralization of the lower extremities begins. Demineralization of the upper extremities has a slower onset. The substantial loss of bone matrix, which also in these cases is paired with loss of muscle mass and strength, highlights the importance of mechanical bone loading.

Q: What stimulus is needed to create bone mass density in adults past the age that is normally associated with peak bone mass?

A: The larger the mechanical load placed on the body, the greater the increase in bone mass density.

A study was made of moderate physical activity that included 200 women between the ages of 35 and 65 over a period of three to four years. Divided into two groups, the test group performing moderate physical exercise for 45 minutes a day, three days a week. The control group was told to be inactive. The control group lost bone mineral density similar to those known for the general population; however, even though those in the moderate physical activity group increased their level of fitness by 13% in the first year of the study, they still had a significant, although slightly smaller bone mass loss than the control group (Smith, et al. 1984). This would indicate that the common low-impact exercises associated with conventional exercise programs for adults and aging adults results in only minimal bone mass density gains.

NASA and Bone Mass Research

In 2005 NASA's Space Life Sciences Division, formerly Life and Biomedical Sciences and Applications, issued a report showing exposure to the microgravity environment of space could negatively impact bone mass at a loss of up to 1% per month. In an effort to learn more about bone mass for the purposes of extended spaceflight, NASA looked at bone mass degradation based purely on the lack of loading on the body. The degradation process seen with individuals on extended space flights resulted from the uncoupling of bone re-absorption and new bone formation and is an acceleration of what is seen in inactive individuals who are experiencing the Earth's gravity Their findings have increased awareness of the importance of mechanical loading for bone remodeling (NASA, 2010). Mechanical loading is the principal action that stimulates osteoblast activity. (Doyle, et al, 1970)

High Levels of Dynamic Loading

Slemenda and other researchers (1991) published a study examining the relationship between bone mineral density and muscular strength in elite junior Olympic weightlifters. The purpose of the study was to better understand the influences of the heaviest types of bone loading on bone mass density. Twenty-five elite junior weightlifters, average age 17.4 years, volunteered for this test, along with a control group of eleven age-matched volunteers of similar height and body mass who were non-weightlifters. As mentioned earlier, younger individuals are able to accept more risk in their exercise routines; therefore, we can look to these individuals, who put the highest levels of load possible on their bodies, to show it is not impact in itself that stimulates osteoblast activity, but rather the load that results from the impact. The average years of training experience for the elite group was 2.7+/-1.4 years in training; the control group had no experience with resistance training. The athletes were recruited from different weight classes according to national ranking and invited to participate in this study. Each of the athletes was among the top 12 junior weightlifters in the United States, according to the national rankings for each weight division in 1989. None of the athletes recorded current or past use of either anabolic steroids or growth hormone, and none had tested positive for such substances in previous athletic competitions leading up to the study. It should be noted that there is no established link between performance-enhancing drugs and bone mass density, though the researchers saw reason to point this fact out with the test subjects. Standard DXA scans were done to determine bone mass density for both the test and control groups in the standard sites for measurement. The results of the DXA scans comparing the two groups showed the weightlifters had an adaptive response of 133% greater bone mass density in the lumbar vertebrae (L2–4) and a 124% greater density in the femoral neck (large bone in the mid thigh). This adaptive response involves the high levels of mechanical loading, but also the strength adaptation, which allows for larger habitual loads to the musculoskeletal structure over time.

Previously, Whalen, et al. (1988) attempted to create a mathematical model that could predict bone reactions to loading based on daily activity loading histories. Most previous studies had gone in different directions, focusing primarily on loading cycles, meaning repetitive non-impact or low-impact activities. The researchers had hypothesized that the bone tissue would remodel, based on daily bone loading maintenance stimulus (activities of daily living). Based on activities and lifestyle, they accurately predicted the bone mass of individuals in the following categories: sedentary, sedentary plus exercise, active, active plus exercise, and athletes. The results of the study showed that the magnitude of loading is a greater influence on bone mass creation, even more so than the number of times the body is loaded. Therefore the larger the load placed on the body, the denser the bone mass will become. The outputs reported were less compelling than with the previous weightlifting study, but only because all activities used as predictors were considered activities of daily living (ADL) or sports activities. No maximal loading was used in this study, as the age groups were wide enough to consider that type of activity as potentially unrealistic, dangerous, or impractical.

Conclusion

The study of Olympic weightlifters showed dramatic differences in bone mass between those who impose large loads on their musculoskeletal system and those who do not. The weightlifters, being competitive, high-performance athletes, regularly perform actions that would be too dangerous for members of the general population. Progressive increases of load over extended periods of time are required for a muscular adaptive response, i.e. greater strength output. Therefore, now the question becomes this: How does an adult induce this progressive increase in loading in order to create greater output from muscular tissue? The next chapter will provide a greater understanding of and solutions to, this question.

CHAPTER 12

PHYSIOLOGICAL BENEFITS

The previous three chapters explained the primary adaptations that can be expected from osteogenic loading:

- **Nervous System adaptations**: Neuro potentiation for momentary explosive strength capability, as well as long-term potentiation for greater muscle fiber recruitment in all activities.

- **Muscular tissue adaptations**: Myofibril development for muscular tissue with increased power-to-weight ratio, as well as accelerated caloric expenditure resulting from increased functional tissue.

- **Bone adaptations**: The osteogenic process that begins as a result of axial mechanical loading being placed on the skeletal system.

The following sections detail the specific physiological benefits that have been seen in individuals from the use of osteogenic loading with the bioDensity device. Primary to all adaptations seen with osteogenic loading is the level of mechanical loading, which approaches or meets the requirements described in earlier chapters regarding multiples of body weight.

Impact Level Loading for the Aging Population

Normative data for the bioDensity Device (bioDensity Server Data, 2011) shows that the 75th percentile Leg Press Load Exposure for females between the ages of 80 to 99 (n=33, mean one year of use) is 612 pounds. This output represents a load many times the typical body weight of a female in this age group.

Impact Level Loading - Sports Performance

Normative data for the bioDensity Device (bioDensity Server Data, 2011) shows the 75th percentile Leg Press Load Exposure for males between the ages of 20 to 29 (n=104, mean one year of use) is 1,974 pounds. This output represents a load many times the typical athlete's body weight.

Neuro-Muscular Adaptation

Using the bioDensity Device, generating load in only the optimal biomechanical positions, users engage a greater amount of muscular tissue than with conventional exercise. This increases the engagement of the CNS and allows for opportunity of momentary muscular failure to occur with both complete myofibril engagement and with the largest potential mechanical load on the body. Significant muscular strength gains can be seen from just a single optimal biomechanical load exposure (Mookerjee, Ratamess, 1999), which is the result of the myofibril development from these sessions of highest force output possible (Zatsiorsky, 2006). The individual skeletal muscles that create the high force output increase myofibril count, which produces a higher power-to-weight ratio in the user, as well as a faster metabolism (more on this in later chapters). A sample of individuals using bioDensity showed an average of 134.5% in force output gain from their experience on bioDensity with an average of one year of use (n=1365, bioDensity Server Data, 2011). Both neurological and muscular tissue effects are applicable for all users, from to high-performance athletes to compromised, elderly individuals: all can greatly benefit from stronger bone tissue and increased muscular strength.

Bone Mass Density Adaptation

User-volunteered unsolicited patient DXA Scans have shown an average 4.5% bone mass gain for individuals in the program for 3 years (n=7, users/patients from initial Napa Valley, CA, test facility). As described in earlier chapters, bone mass degradation does not begin with symptoms; however, either notified by their physician or alerted by a bone fracture, once individuals know their bone mass density is compromised, their self-confidence in physical activity diminishes. With diminishing self-confidence comes a decrease in activity, which thereby further diminishes balance and muscular strength. The individuals with the experience of increased bone mass density can have drastic lifestyle improvements as they can reengage many activities that they had previously abandoned. The increase in potential activity that an individual will reengage in after rebuilding the lost bone mass density is synergistic with many aspects of general health.

Endocrine Adaptation

The hormonal system is stimulated by muscular activity and circulation to secrete anabolic hormones and neurotransmitters that are known to enhance feelings of well being and to reduce stress hormones. As a result of using osteogenic loading, anabolic hormones are enhanced: human growth hormone is multiplied, free testosterone rises, serotonin levels increase, and cortisol is reduced. These endocrine responses help promote balance in the autonomic nervous system and benefit the processes of growth, recovery and regeneration, all of which create an environment for positive change.

CHAPTER 13

BIODENSITY CHEST PRESS

OVERVIEW

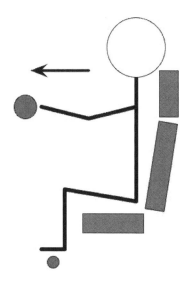

Figure 13-1, bioDensity Chest Press

The figure above shows an individual in a position close to full extension (as detailed, in Figure 10-3 [Chapter 10], the position of optimal biomechanics/impact range). This is the position of loading that provide maximum impact protection.

When an individual falls forward to keep from hitting the ground, the hands are placed in front of the upper body to brace for the impact. This is a reflex of body to protect itself. As this reflex occurs quickly to avoid hitting the head against the ground, the hands come forward and brace for impact, but the positioning will reflexively be the same each time someone falls. You wouldn't see an individual bracing for a fall with completely straight arms, as this may cause an injury. In this scenario, the skeletal structure is bearing all of the loading in an axial manner, thereby having a high risk of injury. An individual would not brace for a fall with the hands just inches in front of the face. The muscles that would be attempting to absorb the impact would be in the weakest possible position, and the attempt to brace for impact would most likely fail.

The bioDensity device adjusts for height of the individual user, as well as the length of the user's arms. The bioDensity exercise movement takes place in this fixed position of approximately a 120° angle. The user monitors the load that they create, on a computer monitor displayed before them. This movement takes the pectorals, triceps, and deltoids to momentary muscular failure in the optimal biomechanical range, which as described in the previous chapters stimulates myofibril muscular growth. Far higher loads are used in this modality, allowing for stimulation of osteoblasts to retain minerals, thereby increasing bone mass density.

CHAPTER 14

BIODENSITY LEG PRESS

OVERVIEW

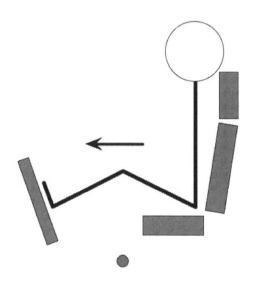

Figure 14-1, bioDensity Leg Press

The leg press, follows the same logic as the chest press and places the legs in a fixed optimal biomechanical position for loading, This position is adjusted to be between 90° and 120°, instead of the 120° angle for the chest press, due to large amounts of tissue compression through the movement. When in movement compression, the user needs to be at the 120° angle. The slight bend of 120° would be the natural position for absorbing impact.

As users create high amounts of load in this movement, the exposure of loading in the optimal biomechanical range is achieved as tissue compression is occurring. The user monitors the load created on the same screen placed in front of him or her. The user presses with the feet and legs to maximize involvement, thereby engaging the quadriceps and calves in the movement. As with the chest press, optimal biomechanical movement of these muscle groups stimulates myofibril muscular growth, as well as osteogenic function in mineral retention.

CHAPTER 15

BIODENSITY CORE PULL

OVERVIEW

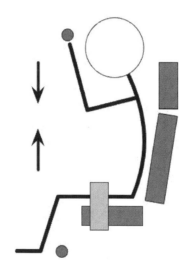

Figure 15-1, bioDensity Core Pull

The core pull mimics the natural motion of going into a fetal position. This movement does not necessarily emulate a position in which an individual would absorb impact' however, this is the natural position an individual takes when protecting the body from damage. The upper body extremities cover the face and head, and the rib cage moves toward the pelvis to protect internal organs. This contracts the abdominal muscles, the obliques. In this movement, the user grasps a bar placed at forehead height, then contracts the biceps, latissimus dorsi (back of the rib cage muscle that pulls the upper arm toward the body), and the entire core in this fetal position. This movement allows for momentary muscular failure in the optimal biomechanical range the biceps, latissimus dorsi, and core.

60-69	*101*	927	1269	1565	2150
70-79	*65*	772	1008	1277	1830
80-99	*22*	579	750	792	1034

Table 17-2, Males Leg Press

Age Group	n=	**Percentiles**			
		25%	**50%**	**75%**	**100%**
20-29	*104*	197	238	286	420
30-39	*101*	187	236	288	449
40-49	*90*	178	246	282	388
50-59	*95*	165	212	275	340
60-69	*101*	162	204	253	307
70-79	*65*	138	176	215	296
80-99	*22*	103	130	143	191

Table 17-3, Males Core Pull

Age Group	n=	**Percentiles**			
		25%	**50%**	**75%**	**100%**
20-29	*104*	376	463	558	918
30-39	*101*	411	478	580	904
40-49	*90*	405	525	548	838
50-59	*95*	369	457	543	748
60-69	*101*	313	418	492	714
70-79	*65*	227	308	392	605
80-99	*22*	135	240	274	428

Table 17-4, Males Vertical Lift

Age Group	n=	**Percentiles**			
		25%	**50%**	**75%**	**100%**

		25%	50%	75%	100%
20-29	82	332	454	585	849
30-39	87	334	420	542	811
40-49	121	322	393	511	947
50-59	201	270	345	428	809
60-69	174	253	306	371	658
70-79	89	186	239	301	490
80-99	33	150	191	221	367

Table 17-5, Females Chest Press

Age Group	n=	Percentiles			
		25%	50%	75%	100%
20-29	82	815	1054	1455	2879
30-39	87	850	1080	1278	2107
40-49	121	779	1052	1275	1851
50-59	201	714	926	1118	1890
60-69	174	600	821	1020	1594
70-79	89	478	577	841	1129
80-99	33	398	560	612	1112

Table 17-6, Females Leg Press

Age Group	n=	Percentiles			
		25%	50%	75%	100%
20-29	82	129	156	182	280
30-39	87	123	161	194	270
40-49	121	124	146	175	259
50-59	201	111	140	166	240
60-69	174	76	111	143	200
70-79	89	81	149	133	191
80-99	33	79	104	120	188

Table 17-7, Females Core Pull

Name: Napa Test Facility, Subject 2
Gender: Female
Age at time of second DXA test: 59
Height: 5'6"
Weight: 170lbs

Medications and supplements taken during bioDensity usage:	
Hormone replacement therapy	No
Testosterone	No
Growth hormone	No
Medications to prevent bone loss	No
Multivitamins	Yes
Calcium supplements	No

Months participating with bioDensity treatment: 24
Number of bioDensity osteogenic loading sessions: 71
(Average .74 sessions per week)
What other physical exercise/fitness activity was engaged concurrently with bioDensity usage? Swimming and yoga once per week.

Highlights:
Bone mass density of the lumbar spine increased by 3.5% from the previous exam. Neck bone mass density increased 3% from the previous exam.

Name: Napa Test Facility, Subject 3
Gender: Female
Age at time of second DXA test: 71
Height: 5'6.5"
Weight: 177lbs

Medications and supplements taken during bioDensity usage:	
Hormone replacement therapy	Yes
Testosterone	No
Growth hormone	No
Medications to prevent bone loss	No
Multivitamins	Yes
Calcium supplements	No

Months participating with bioDensity treatment: 20
Number of bioDensity osteogenic loading sessions: 44
(Average .44 sessions per week)
What other physical exercise/fitness activity was engaged concurrently with bioDensity usage? Dancing and walking.

Highlights:
Bone mass density of the lumbar spine increased by 5% from the previous exam. Femoral bone mass density increased 1% from the previous exam.

Name: Napa Test Facility, Subject 4
Gender: Male
Age at time of second DXA test: 70
Height: 6'4"
Weight: 285lbs

Medications and supplements taken during bioDensity usage:	
Hormone replacement therapy	No
Testosterone	No
Growth hormone	No
Medications to prevent bone loss	No
Multivitamins	Yes
Calcium supplements	No

Months participating with bioDensity treatment: 36
Number of bioDensity osteogenic loading sessions: 62
(Average .44 sessions per week)
What other physical exercise/fitness activity was engaged concurrently with bioDensity usage? Mild bicycling.

Highlights:
This subject had not had a DXA scan for six years. The second DXA scan was administered 36 months after beginning osteogenic loading. From the age of 64 to 70 the patient has not had significant bone mass loss, therefore is not in higher risk of fracture.

Name: Napa Test Facility, Subject 5
Gender: Female
Age at time of second DXA test: 62
Height: 5'4"
Weight: 139lbs

Medications and supplements taken during bioDensity usage:	
Hormone replacement therapy	Yes
Testosterone	No
Growth hormone	No
Medications to prevent bone loss	No
Multivitamins	Yes
Calcium supplements	No

Months participating with bioDensity treatment: 15
Number of bioDensity osteogenic loading sessions: 36
(Average .60 sessions per week)
What other physical exercise/fitness activity was engaged concurrently with bioDensity usage? Aerobics 3 to 4 times a week.

Highlights:
Bone mass density of the lumbar spine increased by 3.4% from the previous exam.

Name: Napa Test Facility, Subject 6
Gender: Female
Age at time of second DXA test: 59
Height: 5'4"
Weight: 125lbs

Medications and supplements taken during bioDensity usage:	
Hormone replacement therapy	Yes
Testosterone	No
Growth hormone	No
Medications to prevent bone loss	No
Multivitamins	Yes
Calcium supplements	Yes

Months participating with bioDensity treatment: 7
Number of bioDensity osteogenic loading sessions: 42
(Average 1 session per week)
What other physical exercise/fitness activity was engaged concurrently with bioDensity usage? Walking on treadmill for 30 min. daily, as well as light weight training.

Highlights:
Bone mass density of the spine increased by 6% from the previous exam. Hip bone mass density had no significant change from the previous exam.

Patient Comments:
"My Bone Density Increased 6%! After years of measurable bone density decline I was desperate to find an answer. Also, for years I have taken non-prescription calcium without any measurable benefit. Then my husband and I read about bioDensity and decided to investigate the system. To my great joy, after only eight months, my latest bone density testing shows a 6% increase. Quite frankly, I would have been happy with no further decline in BMD, but a 6% increase is just over the top. Add to this, I am now stronger and enjoying everything I do more."

Name: Napa Test Facility, Subject 7
Gender: Female
Age at time of second DXA test: 61
Height: 5'3"
Weight: 123lbs

Medications and supplements taken during bioDensity usage:	
Hormone replacement therapy	No
Testosterone	No
Growth hormone	No
Medications to prevent bone loss	No
Multivitamins	No
Calcium supplements	No

Months participating with bioDensity treatment: 18
Number of bioDensity osteogenic loading sessions: 38
(Average .53 sessions per week)
What other physical exercise/fitness activity was engaged concurrently with bioDensity usage? Dance frequently, ride bike and hike.

Highlights:
Bone mass density of the lumbar spine increased, test results show .954 gm/cm² up from .821 gm/cm² a T Score of -0.8 a classification of normal, up from -2.1 which is a classification of osteopenia.

Name: Napa Test Facility, Subject 8
Gender: Female
Age at time of second DXA test: 79
Height: 5'3"
Weight: 129lbs

Medications and supplements taken during bioDensity usage:	
Hormone replacement therapy	No
Testosterone	No
Growth hormone	No
Medications to prevent bone loss	No
Multivitamins	Yes
Calcium supplements	No

Months participating with bioDensity treatment: 24
Number of bioDensity osteogenic loading sessions: 46
(Average .48 sessions per week)
What other physical exercise/fitness activity was engaged concurrently with bioDensity usage? Moderate activity.

Highlights:
Improving from a diagnosis of osteoporosis to a diagnosis of osteopenia. Bone mass density of the lumbar spine increased. Test results show a T Score of -2.1, up from -3.1. There were hip density improvements as well, with a T Score of -1.6, up from -1.8.

CHAPTER 19

OPTIMAL DOSE/RESPONSE FOR

OSTEOGENIC LOADING

The following details the current knowledge of the use of osteogenic loading with bioDensity. In these subsections, research on myofibril hypertrophy, bone mass changes, and sports performance are reported with their relation to osteogenic loading protocols. One of the authors is the inventor/developer of the bioDensity. He and the rest of the authors acknowledge the protocols are based on indications of research with these adaptive responses, but no limitations should be placed on how bioDensity could be applied. Currently two long-term studies are being conducted for application with post-menopausal females and kidney dialysis patients. Potential exists for outcomes to indicate modifications of protocols based on their findings. The authors encourage further testing, research on protocols, and application of bioDensity.

Frequency, How Often Should bioDensity Be Used?

With conventional resistance training, frequency can be on a schedule where stimulation of a muscle group/body part can take place multiple times per week. This is, as stated in earlier chapters, due to the sarcoplasmic adaptive response. In the 1970's Arthur Jones, the founder of Nautilus Corporation and inventor of its products designed a cam system, which the

Nautilus products were all designed around. This cam system was designed to provide variable resistance through a range of motion. Specifically the cam delivered more resistance when closer to the impact range/more extended range, and less resistance in weaker ranges. Jones had observed the uniqueness of the optimal biomechanical/impact position just as was applied in the bioDensity development. He believed that when fully exhausting the muscle from a myofibril standpoint, which would be facilitated by the cam design, that stimulation should only take place one time per week. The reason being that the myofibril adaptation is the development of new functional tissue, and the rate of this occurrence can take far longer than the replenishment of sarcoplasm as with conventional resistance training type exercise. Jones tested his theory with other researchers in the *Spine Journal*, showing that one use of high intensity training, one time per week on an isometric lumbar device, using the optimal biomechanical range was as or more effective than a more frequent protocol (Graves, et al. 1990). Similar observations were made by some of the same researchers the next year that performed a 12 and 20-week analysis on lumbar extension torque (Carpenter, et al. 1991). No more stimulation, with optimal biomechanical range training, than one or two times per week was discussed in another study of a torso rotation device (DeMichele, et al. 1997).

Dr. David Staplin compares the myofibril adaptive response process to wound recovery. He illustrates how the process from stimulus to complete adaptation can vary "from 5 days to over 6 weeks." (Staplin, 1997) This understanding has become an integral part of the bioDensity device software algorithm and is explained in greater depth in appendix A.

Osteoporosis

The largest safe levels of axial-mechanical loading, which approach or match the levels provided by impact, are the most effective for both building and maintaining bone mass density (U.S. Surgeon General, 2004). The protocol of the four osteogenic loading movements, performed one time per week on the bioDensity device is recommended to the majority of users; however, certain aspects and features provided by the bioDensity software aid the individual's effort to achieve the most rapid adaptations. The adjustments of the "Hold Time" allows progress to continue, as this adjustment can enhance the level of comfort and still allow for adaptation. As the individual is asking maximum involvement from the CNS and motor control systems, the CNS cannot be allowed distraction. Any significant level of discomfort can be a distraction to the CNS, hereby compromising motor control and muscular force output.

Loading Hold Times

Adaptation times differ between muscular and bone tissue. Muscular remodeling may take months or years, depending on the individual and the variables in the individual's life. Bone remodeling, however, is more linear. As each new osteoblast emerges from the center of the bond, the migration process begins toward the hardened outer cortex. It is during this time that the osteoblast gathers minerals and becomes a part of a dense structure of minerals with the other osteoblasts. Conversely, bone adaptation is not based on nominal or light axial mechanical loading. This process of the migration to the outer cortex takes longer, and the time grows longer as individuals age, so by its very nature, the bone adaptations take longer to manifest than the myofibril muscular adaptations. Adjusting the hold time can bypass potential discomfort felt in bone tissue and still allow for myofibril muscular adaptation.

The following is a performance report of a 62-year-old female diagnosed with osteoporosis who made this loading hold time change, then continued to make progress by increasing force production:

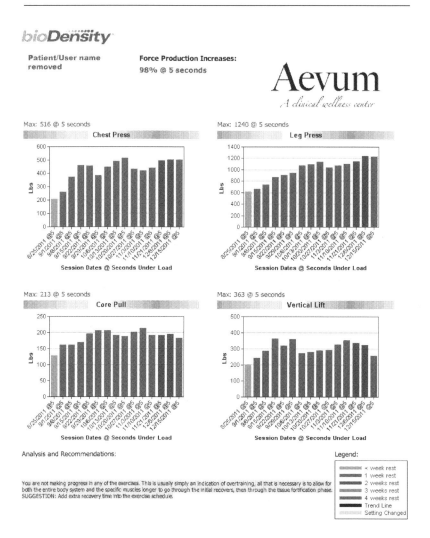

Figure 19-1, Performance Report from osteoporotic user

Comfort Must be Maintained

Unlike conventional exercise, comfort must be maintained throughout the use of bioDensity. As maximal force production requires complete engagement of action potential, nothing that could take away from the engagement of the CNS can be present. This is why bioDensity has the option to use longer hold times for the contractions than the default time of five seconds. With a longer hold time, the individual has the opportunity to build load just short of the point of discomfort, and extra time is taken maintaining this position while at the same time holding for momentary muscular failure to occur.

An example of this would be an individual capable of a 600 pound load in the chest press movement. Over time the individual realizes that discomfort in the hands during the movement is the limiting factor. Momentary muscular failure is not occurring as discomfort is the limiting factor in the movement. This is not the intended stimulus; therefore, something must be done so that momentary muscular failure can occur once again. Increasing the workload and slightly decreasing the intensity of the movement accomplish this, as explained below.

Instead of perceiving discomfort at 600 pounds, the individual may hold a slightly decreased load for an extended period of time, thereby taking longer to get to momentary muscular failure, but still allowing that stimulus to occur. Some users have experienced that, after using a longer holding time for a given movement, they can become comfortable with the load that they were previously not comfortable with, regardless of having to maintain that load for the longer period of time. This could be a reflection of the different times required for adaptation. Myofibril hypertrophy may be occurring at a more rapid rate than the adaptation of bone mass on the basis of force production and comfort. More research is needed analyzing the rates of adaptive response between muscular and bone tissue through the use of bioDensity.

JAQUISH * SINGH * HYNOTE * CONVISER

Muscular Endurance

Muscular endurance is the ability of a muscle to sustain repeated contractions against a resistance for an extended period of time. The standard protocol for training to build muscular endurance depends heavily on cardiovascular training. This optimizes the delivery of oxygenated blood to the target muscle tissue, fueling the tissue for additional contractions. Many athletes training with endurance-type activity engage in little or no conventional resistance training, as holding excess muscular weight via sarcoplasmic adaptation is not desired.

The use of osteogenic loading conversely can have a positive effect on individuals training for muscular endurance. The nature of myofibril hypertrophy is the increase of contractile property within each cell. This means that, for a given amount of work with an individual who is having continued adaptation with the creation of myofibril structures, more receptor sites exist for ATP. The need for ATP, however, does not increase unless the workload increases. With osteogenic loading muscular tissue can become optimized for endurance due to the increased ATP receptor affect of myofibril hypertrophy.

Muscular Power

Soviet sports performance trainers, who used optimal ranges of motion for maximum myofibril engagement, observed that they would specifically narrow the range of motion during training to focus just on the area where an individual is strongest. The theory was to use the place (the range of motion where the athlete is strongest since in that place) the athlete must be using more muscular tissue than in any other given range of motion. These observations were later confirmed (Mookerjee and Ratamass, 1999).

Another sports performance theory that has been tested and proven multiple times is periodization (Plisk and Stone, 2003). Individuals engaging in periodization would stagger certain types of training so that exposures of a certain type would be further apart, as well as scheduling certain exposures or repetition rates with shorter time in between. The following is an example of a periodization schedule:

Week 1: POWER
Monday - Explosive power, all pushing muscle groups (lifts include: bench press, squat)
Thursday - Explosive power, all pulling muscle groups (lifts include: dead lift, bent-over row)

Week 2: VOLUME, 2 pushing days, one pulling
Monday - Lightweight, high repetition pushing muscle groups.
Wednesday - Lightweight, high repetition pulling muscle groups.
Friday - Lightweight, high repetition pushing muscle groups.

Week 3: VOLUME, 2 pulling days, one pushing
Monday - Lightweight, high repetition pulling muscle groups.
Wednesday - Lightweight, high repetition pushing muscle groups.
Friday - Lightweight, high repetition pulling muscle groups.

Week 4: Repeat with Week 1

(The above conventional, periodized resistance exercise program is designed for an athlete who is training for both muscular volume and strength. Other periodized programs can be different, depending on the athlete's goals.)

The reason for this exercise protocol design is primarily acknowledging that the myofibril stimulus is only effective if the proper period of time passes for an adaptive response to occur, before the stimulus is reapplied. Also, the two weeks of volume-type resistance exercise are for the creation of sarcoplasmic development. This means that the goal is to divide different types of stimulus, based on their independent rate of recovery/adaptation. The sarcoplasmic adaptive response requires a much shorter period of time to occur; therefore, the stimulus is repeated at a more rapid rate. Periodization protocols have become popular with high-performance athletic training but are often viewed as both complicated and, as high loads are used in a full range of motion, dangerous to members of the general population who have health as their primary objective. In order for the difference in stimulation type, the "power" days require heavy loads (relative to the individual) in explosive motion movements. This may enable myofibril stimulation, but the risk of injury is increased.

Osteogenic loading can offer the benefits seen with periodization but without many of the drawbacks. Previous to the creation of the bioDensity device, myofibril stimulus was difficult to create and isolated from sarcoplasmic stimulation, as described above. Often, when an athlete would engage in high-intensity resistance exercise, he or she would be stimulating some of each type of development. Osteogenic loading has permitted the complete division of stimulus, thereby allowing for an individual to focus on myofibril development, and sarcoplasmic development at separated intervals that are satisfactory to optimizing results, one independently from the other.

Young Adult, High-Performance Athletes or Aspiring Athletes

Periodization has little to do with a special combination of stimulus and adaptive response or with a rhythm with growth cycles, though it is often discussed in this regard. There is a lack of research indicating a connection or synergy between sarcoplasmic, and myofibril development. Therefore, we must treat each stimulus and adaptive response as separated activities that do not conflict, as is also true of their respective repetition rates (how often an individual engages in each type of activity). Conflicts may be apparent only when the momentary and or immediate recovery from an exercise has not yet taken place before engaging in the other activity. For example, the individual who engages in sarcoplasmic training by lifting conventional weights would not benefit by immediately beginning a myofibril stimulus (high-intensity, explosive weight training, or osteogenic loading/bioDensity) as the conventional session would deplete the fuel stores within the muscle cells (ATP, glycogen, creatine phosphate). This would not allow for a maximal contraction that would be the required for myofibril stimulation. Conversely, if completed in the reverse order, both types of stimulus could be done on the same day, and would not conflict.

The Mechanical Stimulation Must Precede the Biochemical Stimulation

The myofibril stimulation is momentary muscular failure of the mechanical network of myofibrils within sarcomere structures. The failure of the mechanical network sends a signal to the CNS that additional functional tissue is needed. In this mechanical stimulus, a small amount of energy is required for the contraction; therefore, the most readily available fuel source is used, that being ATP. This ATP is replaced within moments of the individual resting by conversion from glycogen. If the individual were to engage in an activity that would create a sarcoplasmic effect as a biochemical function, the effort would not be compromised by the previous activity. There is also evidence that indicates neurological inhibition processes for loading would be altered through bioDensity stimulation via neural potentiation.

Using bioDensity for Neural Potentiation

The bioDensity device can be used for potentiation purpose, meaning that an individual wishing to increase the amount of muscle fiber recruited via the CNS can increase this engagement for a period of time. Short-term explosive force neural potentiation occurs, with the shortest duration and highest resistance maximal voluntary contractions (Bhem, 2004). If an individual chooses to use the bioDensity device for neural potentiation, in order to prepare the neuromuscular system for another activity or event, the engagement of each movement should be maximal; however, the individual must disengage before momentary muscular failure is reached. (Gullich and Schmidtbleicher, 1996, Aagaard, et al, 2002). This amplification can exist 10 minutes following the contraction (Trimble and Harp, 1998). A gymnast, for example, could engage in the vertical lift movement before an event that required explosiveness. This would increase CNS activity, as well as engagement of additional muscular tissue in the explosive activity. Osteogenic loading is one of the few modalities' that can be applied as a preparation for an athletic event, that won't degrade performance in the event. Often on the sidelines of sporting events exercise bikes have been seen, and more recently vibration platforms. These devices are used for similar reasons, simply to increase neuromuscular activity so the athlete has more contractile tissue firing through movement in the actual event.

CHAPTER 20

CALORIC USAGE IMPLICATIONS

WITH OSTEOGENIC LOADING

The dose response protocol for fat loss with osteogenic loading is standard and aligned with the algorithms that recommend the rate an individual uses the bioDensity device. A more specific understanding of cellular usage of calories is principal in understanding how osteogenic loading can aid in the process of fat loss.

The rates at which adults worldwide have become overweight and obese have been escalating. In 2005 Speiser et al determined, 7% of the world population is considered by the medical community to be overweight or obese. Currently of the 6.7 Billion people in the world the WHO (2011) determines that 1.5 billion are overweight or obese. Furthurmore, 65% of the world's population lives in countries where overweight and obesity has a higher mortality than underweight.

Though the restriction of caloric intake is primarily the strategy for body fat reduction, certain exercise programs have been associated with amplification of fat loss when used with restriction of caloric intake. The concept of "weight loss" is not the same as "fat loss." Engaging in osteogenic loading, stimulating a myofibril effect and an increase in bone mass can alter body composition, but not necessarily body weight.

A recent study used intermittent high-intensity conventional resistance exercise to examine fat loss and insulin levels in young females at the University of New South Wales, Sydney, Australia. There were three groups in this study: one using high-intensity conventional resistance exercise, another group that performed moderate-intensity exercise, and a control group that did not exercise. Previous studies had indicated that moderate intensity of exercise led to fat loss ranging from nominal amounts to non-responsive (Shaw, et al. 2006), All subjects selected for this study were of similar BMI and were between the ages of 18 and 30 years. This group was also ethnically diverse as there were 12 Chinese, 18 European, 3 Southeast Asian. and 1 African subject. After the 15 week protocol the high-intensity conventional resistance exercise group had lost an average of over 2 kg in fat mass, which included 1.40 ± 0.17 kg of trunk fat. Both the control group and the moderate intensity exercise group saw nominal gains (<1kg) in fat mass at the conclusion of the study. Given that intensity is the only difference between the groups, discovering the stimulus that could deliver intensity yet increase compliance could make this type of effect acceptable to a larger population base. It should be noted that the researchers cited that many high-intensity protocols prescribed to sedentary, overweight individuals suffer from poor compliance, meaning that the individuals stop following the program. Osteogenic loading provided by bioDensity satisfies this concern and appeals to a larger base.

Exercise physiologists, in an effort to encourage those not engaging in physical activity, often recommend exercise protocols with moderate intensity. The above study shows that this approach is ineffective. Intensity of stimulus is not necessarily associated with whatever activity seems difficult, however. Intensity from a myofibril development standpoint means engaging the largest (in a given movement) number of myofibrils at the point of momentary muscular failure. With osteogenic loading, stimulation occurs in the optimal biomechanical position, thereby ensuring the most intense stimulus to the CNS and, with it, the greatest myofibril adaptive response.

Another study illustrated that the highest intensity of load exposure has the largest synergistic effect with metabolic rates, meaning the number of calories an individual will use in a day (Trapp, 2008). As the group of 78 adolescent males and females (33% of whom were overweight, and 18% were obese) progressed through the experiments, the loads that they were asked to lift would become progressively heavier. This was to potentially match the strength gains the subjects would be experiencing. The protocol was a standard high-intensity conventional resistance training. As with Trapp's study, the subjects had decreasing waist girth, decreases in visceral fat, and increases in strength to weight (power-to-weight) ratio. This would indicate increases in basal metabolic rates. (Benson, Torode, and Fiatarone Singh, 2008)

Muscular Development, for the Acceleration of Fat loss

It has often been suggested that individuals attempting to lose body fat engage in cardiovascular exercise. This activity increases the caloric demands of the body, as the heart, lungs, and other involved muscular tissue all participate in the activity, thereby creating a greater output as a demand from the supporting systems. The individual who engages in cardiovascular activity to promote fat loss is increasing the caloric demand his or her body has during the act of the exercise, as well as in the recovery phase when the body replenishes glycogen and other energy stores in the muscular tissue. After this recovery process has been completed, however, the benefits, from a caloric usage standpoint, stop. To continue receiving benefits from cardiovascular exercise, this activity must be repeated on a regular, even daily basis.

More recently, conventional resistance training has been recommended to accelerate the process of fat loss and was considered superior to cardiovascular exercise. (Ormsbee, et al. 2007). Such a recommendation has appeared on the Oprah Winfrey show, recommending to women that they engage in conventional resistance training, and even commenting that by doing this "you'll lose 40% more fat" (Campbell, 2010). The reason for the recommendation of resistance training relates to the demand the muscle cell/fiber places on the body at all times, not just during the moments of actual exercise and recovery. This is true for both types of muscular development, sarcoplasmic and myofibril, but the process is different. Note the following graphics and explanations associated with each type of development:

Sarcoplasmic Effect, and Metabolism

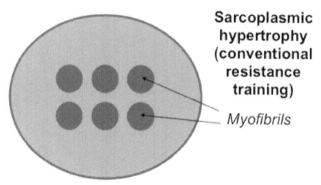

Figure 20-1, Sarcoplasmic hypertrophy

When examining the above image, the sarcoplasmic effect is shown. In the process of accumulating additional sarcoplasm within the individual muscle cell/fiber, the heart has to work harder to pump the blood to the target muscle or group of muscles. The body additionally has to create the elements of the sarcoplasmic expansion of the cell; then after this process is completed, the body reabsorbs the excess sarcoplasm. This process is similar to building a blister. The blister appears as a response to trauma; the fluid within the blister temporarily buffers additional irritation from deeper tissues, and then is reabsorbed into the body. This entire process may take multiple days or even more than a week. This means the activity level as a result of the effect is increased, thereby increasing caloric usage throughout the body, most importantly for a longer period of time after activity then with cardiovascular exercise.

Myofibril Effect, and Metabolism

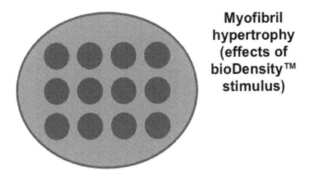

Myofibril hypertrophy (effects of bioDensity™ stimulus)

Figure 20-2, Myofibril hypertrophy

The above depiction of myofibril development shows the process of gaining within a single cell of the individual myofibrils. In actuality, the myofibrils are bundled into sarcomere structures, and this image is a simplification. In the process of developing more myofibrils within sarcomere structures, the central nervous system calls upon free-floating proteins within the sarcoplasm to merge and become these myofibril units. When these units begin to develop and exist within the muscle cell/fiber each individual myofibril generates a caloric demand, as this development is true new tissue growth. The maintenance of all functional tissue has caloric demand, and since when new myofibrils are created, the free-floating proteins used are the replaced with new proteins. The creation of myofibrils is not limited by stores of protein in the muscle cells/fibers, but the potential breakdown of myofibrils is directly related to protein stores (Schimke, 1970). When an individual creates a myofibril response, he or she will keep this functional tissue as long as the protein stores do not diminish. (Such a diminishment typically results from immobility, inability to ingest food, or muscular wasting disease.) The more myofibril development and individual stimulants, the faster metabolism the individual will have. The highlights of metabolic responses to different types of exercise are summarized in the table below:

- Cardiovascular exercise - Increases caloric usage during, and immediately after the exercise event.

- Conventional resistance exercise - Increases caloric usage for multiple days in managing biochemical changes within muscle cells/fibers. In high-intensity form this activity could stimulate a small degree of myofibril response as well.

- High-intensity powerlifting - Increases caloric usage due to a large myofibril adaptation. As long as the individual is able to ingest calories and is not made immobile, the increase in caloric usage can potentially continue for years. Risk of injury is high with this activity.

- Osteogenic Loading with bioDensity - The same or larger increase in caloric usage as seen with high-intensity powerlifting but a greatly reduced risk of injury.

In a 1994 study, 2 men and women aged 56 to 80 years were put through a high-intensity resistance training protocol for 12 weeks, focusing on conventional exercise. However weights selected were 80% of the subjects' one repetition maximum. Though conventional resistance equipment was used, due to its intensity and high loading nature the protocol selected bears more resemblance to high-intensity powerlifting than a typical conventional resistance training protocol for individuals in this age category. The results of this study showed that, after the 12 weeks of the protocol, the energy requirements of the body increased by approximately 15%. The metabolism/caloric requirements that each individual had averaged were 15% greater at the conclusion of this study. The idea that individuals could increase the caloric demand of their bodies by a similar level, then maintain and possibly increase this effect over months and years of their lives—that is the goal osteogenic loading with bioDensity can satisfy.

In focusing on the loading of the body, an individual can increase levels of function and health in multiple organs, as well as improve body composition, by increasing muscle mass and reducing body fat. An individual cannot lose weight with exercise, only with caloric restriction, hence the statement at the beginning of this chapter about the differences between fat loss and weight loss. However, even if an individual does not restrict calories and is engaging in conventional resistance training (or to a greater degree during osteogenic loading with bioDensity), the body composition will change by increasing the amount of muscular tissue and lowering the level of fat in the body. Loss of fat mass in the body is systemic, meaning an individual cannot engage in a type of exercise to reduce the levels of body fat in just one specific area. When body fat levels decrease, the individual gets leaner all over his or her entire body, and specific distributions from one body part to the next compared to other individuals are primarily genetically linked. (Bouchard, Despres, and Maurieg, 1993)

Metabolic Syndrome, and Type II Diabetes

With most deconditioned individuals who are also overweight or obese, the excesses of abdominal fat are deposited as both subcutaneous fat (immediately under the skin) and intra-abdominal fat, a layer under the abdominal muscles, within the abdominal cavity. Individuals with healthy levels of body fat have no or only nominal deposits of intra-abdominal fat. Overweight, and obese individuals begin to deposit fat in this location. These deposits can indicate resistance to insulin, which assists glucose (the building blocks for glycogen, energy in muscle) to enter the cells of the body. In an individual who develops insulin resistance, the body begins to have a diminishing response to insulin, therefore produces increasing levels insulin. As these insulin levels rise, kidney function suffers, and levels of blood fats like triglycerides increase. This results in increased risk for coronary artery disease, stroke, and type II diabetes. The medical community refers to this as "Metabolic Syndrome."

Treating Insulin Resistance/Metabolic Syndrome

Physicians prescribe medications to treat an individual's symptoms of metabolic syndrome; however, the only non-pharmaceutical recommendation is to improve body composition. As described above, this is the process of developing muscular tissue, while at the same time reducing body fat. When an individual engages in a high-intensity conventional resistance-training program or engages in osteogenic loading, the activity focuses on the development of muscular tissue. The differences in caloric demand placed on the body by adipose tissue (fat tissue) are significant: compared to muscular tissue.

- **One pound of adipose tissue burns approximately 2 calories per day.**

- **One pound of muscular tissue burns approximately 6 calories per day.**
(Heymsfield, 2002)

An individual using bioDensity may burn an increased number of calories for each pound of muscle tissue because of the addition of functional inner-cellular structure, the nature of myofibril development.

It is this difference in caloric usage between the two different types of tissue that results in changing body composition. This change decreases body fat levels, including intra-abdominal fat (Hunter, et al. 2002; Cuff, et al. 2003; Tresierras and Balady, 2009). By developing muscular tissue, an increase in insulin receptor sites occurs, as shown in a study of type II diabetes patients (Irvine and Taylor, 2009).

Organ Function

Considering the increases in energy requirements of the body, the synergistic effects of osteogenic loading are greater than just the potential for body fat reduction. The processing of calories to create new functional tissues involves the heart, lungs, digestive organs, liver, and kidneys. Placing increasing demands on these organs forces performance improvements and efficiency throughout the body.

When an individual is deconditioned, he or she often begins to store excess body fat. This result of decrease in activity level is followed by atrophy of muscular tissue (breakdown of the sarcomere structures and loss of sarcoplasm). This decrease may also be paired with increased caloric intake; however, this does not necessarily happen. By lowering the demand for calories within the muscular tissue and maintaining an equal caloric intake, the number of calories the body needs decreases. With the supply of calories remaining constant, adipose tissue/fat will be stored.

CHAPTER 21

DISCUSSION

The development of osteogenic loading, as a concept, did not come from an analysis of existing equipment or devices. The research for osteogenic loading began at the cellular level, looking at muscle, and bone with respective adaptations of each, with this body of research spanning more than 100 years.

Though the modality differs from other modalities in exercise and therapy, the principle of applying a high level of load to the body, which initiates an adaptation, is a concept that has existed for more than 100 years. The osteogenic loading advancement comes from using impact positions in isolation, enabling individuals to deliver multiples of their own bodyweight into the musculoskeletal system. High load in impact has been well understood also, with research showing that gymnastics/jump-landing impacts being that of six multiples of bodyweight (Robinson, et al., 1995, Friedlander, et al. 1995, Heinonen, et al., 1996, Marcus, 1996, Fuches, Baure, and Snow, 2001), levels of loading not possible with conventional resistance training. This type of high impact training has heretofore been considered dangerous, but now through advanced research techniques, an exceedingly large population can use the osteogenic loading stimulus of bioDensity in a safe and controlled manner. Readers are encouraged to review the references cited in this book to gain an even greater understanding of natural impact positions, and the adaptations of the human body with these osteogenic loads.

We encourage the research community to challenge all the assumptions and conclusions in the review of literature within this text. We do not see this document as a final statement on potential solutions for conditions of aging, rather this the first of many research findings that will allow broad groups to use and understand osteogenic loading for improvement of their lives or the lives of their patients/users. Further research, some being conducted now, will bring greater understanding to the benefits of this modality and specific disease states.

GLOSSARY OF TERMS

Cancellous Bone Tissue - This is the sponge-like tissue inside the medullary cavity of the bone where the bone marrow is located.

Compact Bone Tissue - This forms the outer layer of the bone; it is the hardest and most dense part of the bone. This outer part of bone tissue is arranged in canals or tube-like structures called Haversian canals that run parallel to the long axis of the bone. These hardened structures have capillaries and nerve fibers within them.

Concentric Contraction - A contraction where the muscle shortens through a range of motion. With conventional fitness/exercise equipment involves imposing loading on the body, the physical reality of conventional full-range exercise will inherently limit an individual in their ability to use higher (or highest possible) loads. When an individual picks up a free weight such as a barbell, he or she is limited by the capacity to hold, balance and manage the weight as it moves through the range of the exercise.

DXA (dual energy x-ray absorptiometry) Scan - The DXA technology is designed to emit two simultaneous x-ray beams aimed at an individual's hip or spine. The level of absorption of these x-ray beams is used to determine the density of the bone mass.

Eccentric Contraction - A contraction where the muscle elongates through the motion as the action potential is a less than the force or load being applied to it. An example of this would be seen in an individual's ability to lower a given weight or load but not the ability to be able to actually lift or raise that load.

Impact Loading - The loads associated with the body in collision with either the ground or an object. The body assumes by reflex, a position that naturally absorbs impact, this position is known as the optimal biomechanical range.

Lining Cells - Bone cells that cover the entire surface of the bone, these are another type of mature osteoblast cell that regulates calcium and phosphate in the bones.

Momentary Muscular Failure - An occurrence where an individual engaging in an exercise reaches a point in a repetition of the exercise where the target muscles can no longer contract. Most occurrences of momentary muscular failure involve the expenditure of stored energy units (ATP, glycogen, and creatine phosphate), which yield a sarcoplasmic adaptation. When momentary muscular failure occurs due to a mechanical inability to produce, or withstand, additional load, a myofibril adaptation can be achieved.

Myofibril - bundles of parallel protein filaments within muscle cells. The thick protein filaments, called myosin, have a diameter of approximately 15 NM (15 billionths of a meter). The thin protein filaments, called actin, have a diameter of approximately 5 NM (5 billionths of a meter). The arrangement of this bundle is called a sarcomere. The contraction of the muscle causes the sarcomere to shorten by action of the protein filaments.

Myofibril Hypertrophy - This type of muscular growth is a response to the highest possible loading of the neuro-muscluoskeletal system, the amount of myofibrils increases within the sarcomere structures, increasing the density and power-to-weight ratio of a muscle cell.

Optimal Biomechanical Ranges - The range of motion that allows for stimulus to the neuro-musculoskeletal system that meets the requirement of loading the body at the levels provided by high impact training in activity.

Osteoblasts - Bone cells responsible for forming and depositing new bone matrix. Following bone fractures osteoclasts and osteoblasts play important roles in repair. There is a delicate balance that must be maintained between these two cell types. If osteoclasts remove old tissue too fast, there is a net bone loss.

Osteoclasts - Bone cells charged with resorbing bone matrix by dissolving its calcium and phosphate, and releasing it into the bloodstream. Osteoclasts create an acidic microenvironment that is necessary to dissolve bone minerals and to activate the enzymes to break down collagen fibers.

Osteocytes - Bone cells that reside in hollows in the bone matrix. The matrix is filled with fluid and osteocytes are interconnected by finger-like extensions through microscopic tunnels. Osteocytes are believed to be the cells that sense mechanical strain. The signal is either through ionic currents that are induced by detecting fluid flow in the tunnels, or the signal is detected by bone deformation. Osteocytes respond to this strain by sending signals that either cause new bone formation or resorption of existing bone.

Osteogenic Loading - The adaptive growth of new, denser bone mass through axial loading of the musculoskeletal system.

Osteopenia - The diagnosis of low bone mass, without having the bone mass levels be degraded to those of osteoporosis. This is a "pre-osteoporosis" condition.

Osteoporosis - The loss of bone mass, as a result of greater porosity of the bone. This loss occurs from osteoblastic function where the lack of axial mechanical loading or force, being placed on the bone tissue, results in new osteoblasts failing to retain minerals, specifically calcium and phosphate.

Sarcoplasmic Hypertrophy - This type of muscular growth involves the movement of blood into the targeted muscles that are being exercised. This blood flow both delivers oxygen for contractions as well as replaces the fuel for contractions, being glycogen and creatine phosphate.

Subchondral Bone Tissue - This is the smooth tissue that is protected by cartilage, at the ends of the bones.

APPENDIX A

BIODENSITY SOFTWARE AND

HARDWARE DESIGN

Timing and Self-loading

The user is kept in a comfortable position throughout the load exposure. The duration of the load exposure is such that the individual user can build into the load he or she is attempting to overtake (provided it is not the first session). This comfort is, of course, a critical element for user retention. If an individual is not comfortable or has to go through pain to reach a result, he or she will be less likely to continue to participate on a long-term basis. Through multiple sessions the user will notice that the slower he or she enters into the load exposure the greater the chance of performing better, as through the load exposure CNS function has proprioceptive qualities. This simply means the human body does not respond well to instantaneous or jarring style loading from a motor control and balance standpoint.

Loading Origin

With bioDensity the individual does not have load imposed on his or her body by lifting or moving a weight. With bioDensity the individual induces the load on himself or herself. This mechanical creation of load is in a semi-static position of optimal biomechanics, allowing for momentary muscular failure in the optimal range of motion. By allowing momentary muscular failure to happen in this optimal biomechanical range, the following occurs:

As maximum myofibril involvement is enabled at the time of momentary muscular failure in the four separate load exposure exercises, myofibril growth is being stimulated. The loading used is higher than any found with conventional fitness/exercise. In the majority of cases, especially for the lower extremities, individuals will be using loads that are multiples of their own body weight. As discussed in earlier examples of high- impact exercise, multiples of body weight are seen in a heel strike with runners (4 to 6 times body weight). With bioDensity, users will have multiples of their own body weight typically, placed on both upper and lower extremities, as well as the loading of the spine.

Software for the User Experience

Developing the chassis of the device to facilitate this new modality involved understanding of both optimal biomechanics, and mechanical engineering. The physical design only supports the activity, the data gathered and analyzed from this device was what would justify/illustrate the stimulus and adaptive response. Software was developed that would capture and analyze the load exposure data, and at the same time present the data in a way where users would be encouraged during the load exposure by their previous data, as well as given performance data to encourage continued use.

When the user begins a bioDensity session, he or she will sit in the seat and the technician operating the bioDensity device will ask the individual for their username. This is usually the users cellular phone number, or home phone number. After the user is logged in and validated, the device is calibrated to compensate for body weight. Once the first load exposure is engaged, this is the Chest Press, the user has a screen in front of them displaying a circular dial. There are indications on this dial of the current load, the threshold (the place where the load exposure countdown begins) and the previous performance number.

This 'dial and needle for load indication' design was to create visual encouragement for the user in the load exposure. As the users create load through the load exposure they see in real time, sampling at 1000 Hz (sample rate of data acquisition and signal conditioning components) the load they are creating. They see this load and compare on the dial with their timed average performance from the previous session. Thereby attempting to create a load that is higher than the one from the previous session. Assuming myofibril muscular growth happened as an adaptive response from the stimulus in the previous session, the users will be able to create a higher load on a consistent basis, one session to the next. Though the bioDensity prototype was built in 2005, as well as its software for visual encouragement, a study was published by the International Journal of Exercise Science in 2010 testing this theory. In this study researchers used 23 college women aged 19 to 23 years, 11 of which were collegiate basketball players, and 12 of which were untrained. Three types of tests were performed on the test subjects, recording their performances of an isometric contraction of 50° on a modified leg extension fitness apparatus. One test was just verbal encouragement to create the highest loading. The second was both verbal encouragement as well as a visualization of how much load they (the test subject) was creating, displayed in front of them. The third was verbal and pain avoidance, meaning the test subjects were given electrical stimulus to induce pain in the quadricep muscles, the greater the force applied by the test subject the less electrical stimulation and consequently less discomfort. Of the three types of encouragement, the study concluded that verbal and visual together enabled the test subject to have the greatest performance. (Amagliani, 2010) This is the protocol of the bioDensity device. A technician guides the user for compliance to protocol, as well as encouragement verbally. The software provides the visualization of the load exposure therefore providing the opportunity for the highest potential load created by the user.

Elements also seen on the screen include, the hold time of the load exposure, the threshold value, the "Override Threshold" button, the buttons to both progress to the next load exposure, and a "Reset Exercise" button for deleting current load exposures for when protocols were not followed. The screen that the user interacts with during the load exposure is seen below.

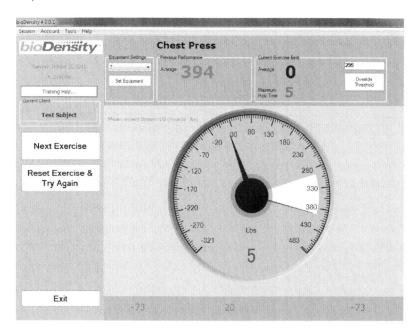

Figure A-1, bioDensity user interface

Hold times are used to ensure safety in each load exposure. As the stimulus required for myofibril muscular development is momentary muscular failure in optimal biomechanical ranges, an assumption can be made that an event that is "momentary" could suffice as a stimulus. Though the stimulus in itself is momentary, the motor/action potential regulation by the CNS requires feedback from pain receptors in a maximal loading event. This feedback process is not instantaneous; therefore event of a load exposure cannot be instantaneous. As the user builds load and here she remains comfortable in the load exposure, higher loads can be attempted.

This is a process where comfort must be maintained and kept by the CNS before continuing. An example of pain/discomfort and feedback would be reaching for a hot stovetop surface. If the individual reaches for a hot stovetop surface, upon nearing the heating element individual will sense the heat through the CNS and will stop moving the hand towards the stove. It is of course possible to ignore the pain/discomfort feedback system by having the same individual slap their hand onto the stove. Obviously the result from this event is a skin burn. If the individual had used the pain/discomfort feedback of the CNS, he or she would have moved to the hand slower in order to gather this information before deciding to either stop moving the hand towards the hot surface, or to continue. With bioDensity the user is required to hold a load for a given period of time, usually this is 5 seconds, but can be advanced based on discomfort levels. In this hold time the user is engaging this process of pain/discomfort feedback. The user begins the load exposure and as the load they create increases, and that they remain comfortable, they can continue to create more loading, until they ultimately reach momentary muscular failure. This hold time mechanism in the bioDensity software both prevents discomfort, and encourages better performance.

To add to the adherence of the user behavior for slow controlled loading through the load exposure, a function called "threshold" was created. The threshold is a number that is chosen as a derivation of the previous performance, and it represents where the load exposure hold time countdown begins. The number is a derivation because the level of difficulty to get to the threshold is different based on each user, as well as the level of development of each user. When a new user account is started, the default thresholds are set for the condition individuals. Therefore when a user first begins treatment with bioDensity records can be created for each of the four load exposures without having to adjust the threshold. At times in later sessions, if a user becomes compromised in joint function, muscular soreness, as well as many potential of the reasons, the threshold can be overridden. Hence the "Override Threshold" button in the software screenshot image above.

Hardware Built for Accuracy and Repeatability

While the patents already issued speak volumes about the unique aspects of bioDensity, the patent applications pending carry its value even further.

One of these patent features includes collecting "Empirical Normative Data", and more specifically doing it via a single database that is connected to every bioDensity machine through the Internet. The "system" aspects of the bioDensity system design was designed with the understanding that users of the system will provide the most accurate exercise data every collected, and will themselves verify the results through weekly sessions, and seeing the progress accurately reported on their individual progress chart. Not only is the weekly session progress reported accurately, but also the user over time realizes that bioDensity works and works well. This realization comes from becoming stronger, being able to do certain activities with more ease, and in the extreme having their Physician provide them with their latest DXA results showing an increase of bone mineral density.

It has always been the case that when selecting the method of normative empirical recording for an object of study, is it possible to study empirically the factual activities or product that is the object of study, or simply collect both the facts/data and evaluations/results from participating evaluators? At the earliest point in the bioDensity design effort it was decided that if the system is to be used by individuals over decades, it must measure accurately the force applied with each exercise, and to record those measurements accurately.

The approach taken removes any element of variation in the exercise data collection. All machines utilize a common system application that interacts with each machine no matter where it is located on the network. While the bioDensity user interface is designed to offer various languages, and two load measurement systems it nonetheless maintains a high level of accuracy.

The accuracy and repeatability are necessary if the measured facts and the user evaluations are to connect properly. When defining the group of people who would likely take part in the bioDensity sessions, and how the recording of machine facts and user evaluations, the selection was somewhat self-evident, particularly since the design objective was to eliminate machine variability, and user feedback variability. All applied force is recorded by Load Cells that are accurate within the range of +/- 1 to 2 % of indicated load. While accuracy is important it is also important to have a repeatable system because the incremental progress over a decade or two by individual users must be able to display the small changes with respect to the user's progress.

Eliminating user variability is driven by the following:

- The design decision was made early on the bioDensity users would never be subject to interrogation methods as it relates to their exercise sessions and the force values they produced, but rather Algorithms would be used to evaluate a particular session's results relative to all prior session results. In this manner any day-to-day subjective reaction to a particular session is eliminated. Since 2005 all bioDensity users have paid for the privilege of using the system, and it was believed that if the users were not receiving sufficient value they would stop paying and using the bioDensity system. A decision to stop is certainly more objective that any session-by-session reaction.

- To further eliminate user variability as it relates to their opinion about their exercise session the bioDensity system was designed to provide a real time printout of the exercise session just completed, and that permits the user to discuss the algorithm comments section of the report or any other aspect of the session with an advisor who is in control of the bioDensity machine. The printed report has the effect of providing the user with "hard" feedback along with the opportunity to discuss progress either positive or negative.

Traditional fitness equipment provides little or no session results, which leaves the user simply sweaty and sore, but not knowing what happened or if it was beneficial. In the case of bioDensity the user knows the data was collected accurately and that the results are understandable. This combination has allowed the collection of Empirical Normative Data that has never been collected before.

By way of illustration, the bioDensity database contains the exercise data of over 19,000 users. This data represents the largest body of "highly accurate" exercise data ever assembled, and it is growing larger every day.

After seven years of collecting empirical data, bioDensity has successfully eliminated the two greatest risks to the value of its database. The machine data was not collected by observations, but rather by accurate and repeatable precision digital load recording, and the user data was not collected by user interrogation or questionnaires.

All of the bioDensity machine and user data/information is reliable, and accessible to researchers who demonstrate how it will be used, and are willing to be subject to normal data use agreements.

Monitoring Adaptation

Sarcoplasmic muscular development happens as a result of circulation and blood demand to target muscular areas during an exercise. This process can be repeated for additional adaptation at a rate provided the time allowed for replenishment of glycogen, and flushing of lactic acid. This is different from each individual, but may be between 48 hours and 96 hours on average. With myofibril development the process of adaptation is very different. The process involves the development of the new functional tissue. New myofibrils in sarcomere structures are developed with in fibers/cells thereby increasing the density of the cells. The development of new functional tissue takes a greater amount of resource from the body then the process of glycogen replenishment. The limitations on the speed of this process have less to do with diet (dietary habits can be optimized to facilitate sarcoplasmic development) and more to do with the body's ability to process the nutrients required to build this new tissue.

No matter what an individual does from a physical fitness/health standpoint enhancing the capacity for developing new living tissue as a consistent rate. Just as an example: No matter how healthy an individual is, eating more vegetables, sleeping more, cutting out unhealthy habits, etc. will not force an individual to grow their fingernails faster. This means, there is a given rate that an individual has for myofibril development, and little can be done to enhance the speed of this process which means the correct amount of time must pass before the adaptive response has taken place and an individual must stimulate again for continued development. Though no differentiation was made in the different types of development, Dr. David Staplin presents this clearly in his 1997 paper comparing this process to wound recovery. He illustrates how this cycle of stimulus to full recovery can vary "from 5 days to over 6 weeks." (Staplin, 1997)

The bioDensity software utilizes algorithms to determine the correct time interval that a user should be returning and attempting another load exposure session. The default, or starting point for each new user is one week. This means when a user begins bioDensity treatment, they must wait at least one week before attempting their second load exposure session. The more sessions a user completes, the more data sets the software has to make recommendations based on. The recommendations, when determined can add an extra week between sessions, thereby having the user use the bioDensity device once every other week. Users will be recommended to return anywhere from one time per week to allowing up to three weeks in between the sessions.

Network Design

As this type of therapy/exercise was new in 2005, collecting as much data as possible was a primary objective. Added to that, as other locations would come online collecting the data and aggregating this data was also a primary objective. As this new modality of therapy/exercise would grow, multiple locations would have it available, and these locations would need to be compliant with set protocols, IE: They all must use the device in the correct way. Adherence to the set protocols was made possible by designing the device to be an Internet appliance. This means that it operates as part of a network only, never independent. Without the connection to the bioDensity server, the device does not function. The design of the bioDensity network has two overarching principals:

Security in Server Side Design

No bioDensity location will have to hire extra IT staff, or have employees that are charged with the responsibility of backing up systems, housing data, or managing data in any way. The bioDensity network works like a wireless phone carrier, an individual will turn their phone on to make a call, and the network is there.

- All data is saved server side, managed and analyzed and available anytime, at any location for both viewing and management.

- Patients/Users automatically receive their performance report in their email sent from the bioDensity server once they have completed their force production session.

Global Database Synergy

By using bioDensity, a location is leveraging a collection of 400,000 force production data points, with a user base of 22,000 individuals. The algorithms that dictate the repetition rate of force production sessions are in perpetual modification. The updates are based on recorded data points of age group and cross-referenced with exercise, activity, and related pharmacological factors.

- Patients/Users will be seeing benefit of predictive software analysis of each force production, with suggestions and guidance for subsequent sessions.

- The longer Patients/Users are engaged the more data is analyzed and the greater benefit they will see.

- Custom branding for locations shows on performance reports. If Patient/User is a guest at another facility and uses a bioDensity device there, the facility branding still shows.

This architecture allowed for data to be captured at the Napa Valley, California test facility without fail. Before moving out of the prototype phase and into production of the device, 40,000 load exposures were recorded by 449 users.

APPENDIX B

FREQUENTLY ASKED QUESTIONS

Through the development of bioDensity, many questions were presented to the researcher regarding application of this new modality of therapy/exercise to the lives of the elderly, busy professionals, and sports performance athletes.

"How is this different from regular fitness training for my bones?"

Loading, multiples of body weight creates the difference.

A study was conducted on weight bearing and muscle loading in respect to bone mineral accrual in pre-pubescent 10 to 13-year-old females, and then reassessed after two years. Out of the 258 females in the study, the average total body bone mass change was an increase of 35+/-9%. The researchers observed that in this impact the mechanical loading on the musculoskeletal structure could be as high as between four and nine times body weight. There is no safe protocol with conventional fitness apparatus in which exercising individuals would be able to use loads between four and nine times greater than their own body weight (Wang, et al. 2007). With bioDensity this magnitude of loading is made possible while still maintaining safety, even for the elderly. According to the bioDensity normative data, females over the age of 70 generated 478 pounds in the 25th percentile, 577 pounds in the 50th percentile, 841 pounds in the 75th percentile, and 1129 pounds in the 100th percentile in the leg press load exposure (bioDensity Normative Data server query, 2011). According to the United States Center for Disease control, the average female between 60 and 74 years of age weighs 147+/-1.2 pounds (Ogden, et al. 2004). This indicates that even the females over 70 in the 25th percentile are using more than three times their own body weight in this load exposure, and those closer to the 75th percentile are using a multiple of 5.7 times their own body weight. This device is providing the stimulus of bone mass that these older females are receiving in the study, without the risks of impact.

"I have joint problems. Is this a contraindication for bioDensity use?"

No. The bioDensity stimulus is all self-induced loading; therefore, the chances of irritating any part of the body, joint, bone, or other body part is low. The potential from injury with bioDensity is diminished from conventional exercise or most other types of physical activity due to its self-loading nature.

"Is there any pain associated with a bioDensity session?"

No pain or discomfort should ever be associated with a bioDensity session or any individual osteogenic load exposure on the bioDensity device. Discomfort during a movement subconsciously distracts the individual, thereby compromising the CNS action potential function. Examples of this are seen in individuals who ignore the hold time function of the bioDensity software and enter into load exposures in an instantaneous or explosive manner. This jarring activity is not comfortable; pain receptor nerves in bone tissue, tendon tissue, and ligament tissue become irritated, and motor control is thereby compromised. The faster or more carelessly an individual enters into a bioDensity movement, the worse he or she will do. As a result of lower loading levels, neither myofibril muscular or skeletal density adaptation will take place to the fullest possible degree, as the stopping point of the action is discomfort, instead of momentary muscular failure.

"I have had back injuries and/or surgeries before. Will this prevent me from using the bioDensity device?"

As with all exercises followed by surgery, this system should only be used with a physician's approval.

"Can I still go to the health club for conventional resistance training/exercise?"

Yes. The osteogenic loading stimulation creates myofibril hypertrophy, whereas conventional weight lifting creates sarcoplasmic hypertrophy. Sarcoplasmic hypertrophy is movement of blood into the targeted muscles. This effect may aid in recovery when using the bioDensity system. It is advisable, however, that, if an individual were planning on using the bioDensity device and on the same day doing conventional resistance training, the bioDensity stimulus should come before the resistance training session. The reason for this order is that adenosine triphosphate (ATP) stores in the myofibrils must be populated. A conventional resistance training session would deplete myofibrils of the needed energy in its most usable form, which is ATP. By doing a bioDensity session first, a very small amount of ATP would be used, but the additional fuel sources of glycogen and creatine phosphate would remain intact. Momentary muscular failure takes place in a sarcoplasmic stimulus when fuel stores are depleted, meaning first ATP, then glycogen and creatine phosphate. The myofibril stimulus requires the most readily available energy, that being ATP.

"Should I continue doing cardiovascular exercise?"

Yes. Cardiovascular exercise is separate from the bioDensity system. The stimulus that bioDensity provides does not directly impact cardiovascular function or performance. Nevertheless, some compelling observations have been made from users at various locations recognizing their perceived cardiovascular performance has increased since beginning the osteogenic loading protocol.

"Does age affect one's ability to use the bioDensity system?"

No. User's ages at the initial Napa Valley test facility ranged from as young as 11 years to as old as 90. . Earlier research had suggested that prepubescent children should not participate in conventional resistance exercise; however, more recent studies have shown positive outcomes in developing prepubescent study subjects. At the Department of Human Performance and Fitness at the University of Massachusetts in Boston, a study was performed to analyze different resistance training protocols on muscular strength in children. Study subjects included 11 females and 32 males between the ages of 5.2 years and 11.8 years. The observations made relevant to this discussion had mostly to do with the children's lack of ability to control the heaviest resistances through a full range of motion (Faigenbaum, et al. 1999). The exercising group saw positive strength outcomes. The study recommends that prepubescent children use lighter weights to safely balancing and controlling movement; however, the issue of balancing and controlling a weight or resistance through range of motion is not relevant with the bioDensity experience. Also, as Wang, et al. (2007) shows, impact-type activities in which prepubescent children engage delivers loading between four and nine times the child's own body weight. The osteogenic loading stimulation from bioDensity provides is only providing this level of loading in a controlled environment.

"I am a woman; will I get bulky?"

No, "bulkiness" comes from sarcoplasmic hypertrophy. This effect moves blood through the muscle cells primarily to deliver oxygenated blood to the target area. After this blood displacement dissipates, the effect leaves a residual of proteins, glycogen, creatine phosphate, minerals, and other components, creating sarcoplasmic effect. With the bioDensity device, the user is only stimulating myofibril development, which is functional and carries little size.

"Will this technology make me lose weight?"

The only thing that will force an individual to have a declining body weight over time is by taking in fewer calories than the amount being used by the body. When an individual begins the bioDensity protocol, he or she is stimulating myofibril development. As previously stated, this is the creation of functional tissue, and functional tissue has an added caloric demand. This makes an individual have a higher resting metabolic rate, thereby increasing the number of calories used by the body through the course of a normal day. As long as the individual engaging in the protocol is consuming fewer calories than this new increased resting metabolic rate amount, body mass will decline.

"Can a women use this device while pregnant?"

While exercise is generally recommended, each woman should consult her physician before using the bioDensity device.

"How accurate is the bioDensity device?"

The bioDensity device measures the output of the movement to measurement devices. Strain guages, also known as the load cells, are used to measure the loading that is created by the user. These measurement devices have a nominal margin of error and are extremely accurate. A user can expect that load exposures performed in different locations will correlate together. This is because of the repeatability of the load exposure events, even on different fixtures. The load cells sample data and process this data into the bioDensity server network at a rate of 1000 Hz.

"What data do you show physicians to confirm increase in progress?"

Physicians can study performance reports that confirm the bioDensity device increases force production/muscular strength, as well as confirm high loads that may even include multiples of body weight, which could indicate the chance of increases in bone mass density. The performance report includes data from each individual movement represented in bar graphs, which the user and physician can analyze. This performance report contains the start date, report date, and the algorithm-driven analysis and recommendations.

"What is the earliest time frame measurable result to detect bone density increase?"

Results depend on each individual user. Pre-and post-DXA scans have been taken by users at the initial Napa Valley test facility have left less than a year in between scans and showing a positive outcome. Once beginning bioDensity therapy, a user should inquire with his or her physician to determine when to next test bone mass density.

"How does this machine help patients with hip or knee replacements?"

The device will help increase muscular strength and build supporting structure around the compromised joint (myofibril muscular development), and improve bone mass, and build the supporting structures of tendons and ligaments as tissue. Due to there being no weights lifted, there is no load imposed on the body that could further irritate the hip and knee replacement. A physician should be consulted who is familiar with the particular joint replacement before engaging in osteogenic loading with the bioDensity device.

"How does this device help patients/users with arthritis?"

Osteoarthritis is the pain and physical limitations that manifest as a result of degradation in protective tissues between bones. Protective layers, such as cartilage, exist so that the bones can move together in comfort. Throughout life individuals can misalign these bones and thereby damage these protective layers. As a degenerative disease, osteoarthritis shows degradation of tissue over time, with many degrees of severity. There are a number of medications primarily focused on the reducing perceived pain of this disease, as well as anti-inflammatory medications, all of which have negative side effects. However, studies have shown that after improving the supporting structure around the affected joint (building the tendons, ligaments, and muscular tissues), the joint action then causes less pain to the individual.

"Reduced joint movement may result in less pain during and after the resistance training" (Topp, et al. 2002). As a study examining dynamic versus isometric resistance on adults with osteoarthritis of the knee, this randomized clinical trial compared the results of 16 weeks with three groups: one group using isometric resistance, another using conventional resistance exercise, and the control group. The measures of this study examined Activities of Daily Living (ADLs) in the time it took to complete daily tasks (such as ascending a flight of stairs and getting up from the floor) and showed that the rate at which these groups were able to complete the tasks determined their comfort/pain levels in the performance of the task. The time it took to complete the tasks with the isometric group decreased by 16% to 23%, and for the conventional resistance exercise group decreased by 13% to 17%. The isometric hold used in this experiment kept knee flexion at 10°, this joint angle was calculated from the foot, in contrast to joint angles due to where the origin of the angle is considered. Those earlier studies were calculated from the hip joint as opposed to from the foot. This means the individuals engaging in the isometric protocol were exposing load at a position where the target muscle tissue (quadriceps) was in a fully contracted position, while at the same time allowing for continued mechanical leverage. This is the position of optimal biomechanics, exactly the principal of osteogenic loading/bioDensity. This kind of loading will improve the condition of a joint and comforting movement for an individual with osteoarthritis. Not only is the user able to develop supporting structure around the compromised joint, but through the process of bioDensity treatment comfort is maintained through the osteogenic movements.

Rheumatoid arthritis is an autoimmune condition that has similar side effects to osteoarthritis, however bears no significant causal relationship. Tendon, ligament, and muscular supporting structure can reduce friction within the joint that in theory would assist in the reduction of pain through ADLs. More research is required with rheumatoid arthritic patients and bioDensity for substantive conclusions.

Lawlor, D.A., Davey Smith, G., & Ebrahim, S. (June 2004). Commentary: The hormone replacement-coronary heart disease conundrum: Is this the death of observational epidemiology?" *International Journal of Epidemiology,* 33 (3): 464–7. PMID 15166201.

Leblanc, A., Schneider, V., Evans, H., Engelbretson, D., & Krebs, J. (1990). Bone mineral loss and recovery after 17 weeks of bed rest. *Journal of Bone and Mineral Research.* 5,8. 1523-4681. 10.1002/jbmr.5650050807

Marcus, R. (1996). Skeletal Impact of Exercise. *The Lancet.* November 1996. 384(9038): 1326-1327.

McGuff, M. D. (2003). Recovery. *Ultimate Exercise Bulletin.* 1(11).

McKenzie, D. K. & Gandevia, S. C. (1987). Influence of muscle length on human inspiratory and limb muscle endurance. Respiration Physiology 67, 171-182.

Mookerjee, S., & Ratamess N. (1999). Comparison of Strength Differences and Joint Action Durations Between Full and Partial Range-of-Motion Bench Press Exercise. Journal of Strength and Conditioning Research, 1999, 13(1), 76–81 1999 National Strength & Conditioning Association.

Most Americans don't exercise regularly. (April 07, 2002). CNN Health. Retrieved from http://articles.cnn.com/ 2002-0407/health/americans.exercise_1_vigorous-activity-leisure-time-exercise-activity-at-least-three?_s=PM: HEALTH; last accessed 21 June 2011. (D7 Study).

Mundy, G. R. Bone remodeling. In: Primer on the metabolic bone diseases and disorders of mineral metabolism, M. J. Favus (ed.), Philadelphia: Lippincott Williams & Wilkins, pp. 30-38. 1990.

National Aeronautics and Space Administration (2010). *Weak in the Knees - The Quest for a Cure.* Washington D.C.. Record created: 2005-02-18T13:15:40-5:00. Reviewed, 2010. Retrieved from http://weboflife. nasa.gov/currentResearch/currentResearchGeneralAr chives/weakKnees.htm; last accessed 02 March 2011.

National Center for Biotechnology Information (2010). *Osteoporosis Thin Bones.* Bethesda, MD: U.S. National Library of Medicine. Last reviewed: January 4, 2010. Retrieved from:http://www.ncbi.nlm.nih .gov/pubmed health/PMH0001400; last accessed 20 February 2011.

Ogden, C.L., Fryar, C.D., Carroll, M.D., & Flegal, K,M. (2004) *Mean Body Weight, Height, and Body Mass Index,* United States 1960–2002. Advance Data from Vital and Health Statistics. 347:1-20.

Ormsbee, M.J., Thyfault, J,P.. Johnson, E.A., Kraus, R.M., Myung, D.C.. & Hickner, R.C. (2007). Fat metabolism and acute resistance exercise in trained men," *Journal of Applied Physiology,* vol. 102, no. 5, pp. 1767–1772.

Petrella, J, K.,, Kim, Jeong-su,, Mayhew, D. L., Cross, J. M., & Bamman, M.M. (2008). Potent myofiber hypertrophy during resistance training in humans is associated with satellite cell-mediated myonuclear addition: a cluster analysis. *Journal of Applied Physiology.* 2008; 104:1736-1742, 2008.

Plisk, S. & Stone, M. (2003). Periodization Strategies. *Strength & Conditioning Journal.* V25, 1524-1602.

Ralston. Stuart H. (2005). Genetic determinants of osteoporosis. *Current Opinion in Rheumatology.* July 2005 - Volume 17 - Issue 4 - pp 475-479.

Rector, R.S., Rogers, R., Ruebel, M., & Hinton, P.S. (2008). Participation in road cycling vs. running is associated with lower bone mineral density in men. *Metabolism Clinical and Experimental.* February 2008. 57(2): 226-32. ISSN: 0026-0495.

Robinson, T. Snow-Harter, C. Taaffe, D. Gills, D. Shaw, J. Marcus, R. (1995). Gymnasts exhibit higher bone mass than runners despite similar prevalence of amenorrhea and oligomenorrhea. *Journal of Bone and Mineral Research.* Jan;10(1):26-35.

Robinson, R, Krzywicki, T., Almond, L., Al–Azzawi, F., Abrams, K., Iqbal, S., & Mayberry, J. (1998). Effect of a low-impact exercise program on bone mineral density in Crohn's disease: A randomized controlled trial. *Gastroenterology.* 115:36-41.

Schimke, R.T. (1970). Regulation of protein degradation in mammalian tissues. *Mammalian Protein Metabolism,* Vol. IV. H. N. Munro, ed., New York, NY. Academic Press,177–228.

Shaw, K., Gennat, H., O'Rourke, P., & Del Mar, C. *The Cochrane collaboration. Exercise for overweight or obesity.* Cochrane Database System Review 2006; 4: 1–88.

Simkin, A., Avalon, J., Leichter, I. (March 1987). Increased trabecular bone density due to bone-loading exercises in postmenopausal osteoporotic women. *Calcified Tissue International*: 59-63.

Slemenda, C. W., Miller, S. L., Hui, T. K., Reister, C. C., & Johnston, J. R. Role of physical activity in the development of skeletal mass in children. *Journal of Bone Mineral Research.* 6:1227-1223, 1991.

Smith, E., Smith, P.E., Ensign, C. J., & Shea, M. (1984) Bone involution decrease in exercising middle-aged women. *Calcified Tissue International.* 1984;36 Suppl 1:S129-38.

Speiser, P.W., Rudolf, M.C.J., Anhalt, H., Comacho-Hubner, C., Chiarelli, F., & Elakim, A. (2005). Consensus statement: childhood obesity. *Journal of Clinical Endocrinology and Metabolism,* 2005; 90: 1871–1887.

Staplin, D. (1997). Understanding recovery: A wound healing model". Retrieved from *Exercise Certification*.com. Last accessed: 05-15-2011.

Sundar, S., Ausk, B. J., Prasad, J., Threet, D., Bain, S. D., Richardson, T. S., & Gross, T. S. (2010). *Rescuing Loading Induced Bone Formation at Senescence.* Seattle, Washington: Department of Orthopedics and Sports Medicine, University of Washington. Sept;2010(6). 9:1-16

Surgeon General (2004). *Bone health and osteoporosis: A report of the Surgeon General.* Rockville, MD. : U.S. Dept. of Health and Human Services, Public Health Service, Office of the Surgeon General ; Washington, D.C.: U.S. G.P.O., 2004. p.436, 223

Taube, W. (2011). What trains together, gains together: strength training strengthens not only muscles but also neural networks. *Journal of Applied Physiology* 111: 347-348, 2011. First published 9 June 2011; doi:10.1152/japplphysiol.00688.2011.

Trapp, E.G., Chisholm, D.J., Freund, J, & Boutcher, S.H. (2008). The effects of high-intensity intermittent exercise training on fat loss and fasting insulin levels of young women. . *International Journal of Obesity.* (Faculty of Medicine, University of New South Wales, Sydney, Australia). 2008, 32, 684–691.

Tresierras M.A., & Balady, G,J. (2009). Resistance training in the treatment of diabetes and obesity: mechanisms and outcomes. *Journal of Cardiopulmonary Rehabilitation and Prevention*, vol. 29, no. 2, pp. 67–75.

Trimble, M.H., 7 Harp, S.S. (1998). Postexercise potentiation of the H-reflex in humans. *Medicine and Science Sports and Exercise.* 30: 933-941.

Topp, R., Woolley, S., Hornyak, J., Khuder, S., 7 Kahaleh, B. (2002). The Effect of Dynamic versus tsometric tesistance training on pain and functioning among adults with osteoarthritis of the knee. *Archives of Physical Medicine and Rehabilitation.* 2002,38;1187-1195

Tsuzuku, S., Shimokata, H., Ikegami, Y., Yabe, K., & Wasnich, R.D. (2001). Effects of high versus low-intensity resistance training on bone mineral density in young males. *Calcified Tissue International.* 68(6):342-347.

U.S. Food and Drug Administration (2010). *Bisphosphonates (marketed as Actonel, Actonel+Ca, Aredia, Boniva, Didronel, Fosamax, Fosamax+D, Reclast, Skelid, and Zometa) Information*, MD: FDA Drug Saftey Communication: October 13, 2010. Retrieved from: http://www.fda.gov/Drugs/DrugSafety/Postmarket DrugSafetyInformationforPatientsandProviders/ucm10 1551.htm.

U.S. Food and Drug Administration (2007). *Evista Medication Guide*, ID: Eli Lilly and Company: Retrieved from: http://www.fda.gov/downloads/Drugs/DrugSafety/ucm 088593.pdf; last accessed 29 February 2011.

Verhoshanski, Y. (1967). Are depth jumps useful?. *Track and Field* 12:9, Translated in: Yessis Review of Soviet Physical Education and Sports 4: 28-35, 1968.

Wang, Q., Alen, M., Nicholson, P., Suominen, H., Koistinen, A., Kroger, H., & Cheng, S. (2007) Weight-bearing, muscle loading and bone mineral accrual in pubertal girls - A 2-year longitudinal study. *Bone, the Journal of the International Bone and Mineral Society.* 40:1196-1202.

Whalen, R. T., Carter, D.R., & Steele, C. R. (1988). Influence of physical Activity on the Regulation of Bone Density. *Journal of Biomechanics*, Vol. 21. No IO. pp. X25-837, 1988.

Whedon, G. D. (1984). Disuse osteoporosis: physiological aspects. *Calcified Tissue International.* 1984;36 Suppl 1:S146-50.

Wilson, G., Elliott, B., & Kerr, G. (1989). Bar path and force profile characteristics for maximal and submaximal loads in the bench press. *International Journal of Sports Biomechanics.* 5:390–402.

Wilson, G. (1994). Strength and power in sports. In: *Applied Anatomy and Biomechanics in Sports*. J. Bloomfield, T. Ackland, and B. Elliott, eds. Boston, MA: Blackwell Scientific Publications, pp. 110–208.

World Health Organization. *Obesity and overweight,* Fact sheet 311. With *Key Facts*. Geneva, Switzerland.: WHO publication, March 2011. Retrieved from: http://www.who.int/mediacentre/factsheets/fs311 /en/index.html, 7 May 2011.

Wolff, J. (1892). *Das Gesetz der Transformation der Knochen*. Berlin, Germany; Verlag von August Hirschwald.

Zatsiorsky, V. Science and practice of strength training. Champaign, IL: *Human Kinetics*, pp. 63-65. 2006.

15500270R00106

Made in the USA
Charleston, SC
06 November 2012